Future of Advanced Registered Nursing Practice

Guest Editor

ROBIN DONOHOE DENNISON, DNP, APRN, CCNS, CEN, CNE

NURSING CLINICS OF NORTH AMERICA

www.nursing.theclinics.com

Consulting Editor
SUZANNE S. PREVOST, PhD, RN, COI

June 2012 • Volume 47 • Number 2

SAUNDERS an imprint of ELSEVIER, Inc.

W.B. SAUNDERS COMPANY

A Division of Elsevier Inc.

1600 John F. Kennedy Blvd., Suite 1800 • Philadelphia, PA 19103-2899

http://www.theclinics.com

NURSING CLINICS OF NORTH AMERICA Volume 47, Number 2
June 2012 ISSN 0029-6465, ISBN-13: 978-1-4557-3899-1

Editor: Katie Hartner
Developmental Editor: Donald Mumford

Nursing Clinics of North America (ISSN 0029-6465) is published quarterly by Elsevier Inc., 360 Park Avenue South, New York, NY 10010-1710. Months of issue are March, June, September, and December. Periodicals postage paid at New York, NY and additional mailing offices. Subscription price per year is, $144.00 (US individuals), $360.00 (US institutions), $260.00 (international individuals), $440.00 (international institutions), $210.00 (Canadian individuals), $440.00 (Canadian institutions), $79.00 (US students), and $129.00 (international students). To receive student/resident rate, orders must be accompanied by name of affiliated institution, date of term, and the signature of program/residency coordinator on institution letterhead. Orders will be billed at individual rate until proof of status is received. Foreign air speed delivery is included in all *Clinics* subscription prices. All prices are subject to change without notice. **POSTMASTER:** Send address changes to *Nursing Clinics*, Elsevier Health Sciences Division, Subscription Customer Service, 3251 Riverport Lane, Maryland Heights, MO 63043. **Customer Service: Telephone: 1-800-654-2452** (U.S. and Canada); **1-314-447-8871 (outside U.S. and Canada). Fax: 1-314-447-8029. E-mail: journalscustomerservice-usa@elsevier.com** (for print support) and **journalsonlinesupport-usa@elsevier.com** (for online support).

Nursing Clinics of North America is covered in *EMBASE/Excerpta Medica, MEDLINE/PubMed (Index Medicus), Social Sciences Citation Index, Current Contents, ASCA, Cumulative Index to Nursing, RNdex Top 100,* and Allied Health Literature and International Nursing Index (INI).

Printed in the United States of America.

Contributors

CONSULTING EDITOR

SUZANNE S. PREVOST, PhD, RN, COI
Associate Dean, Practice and Community Engagement, University of Kentucky, Lexington, Kentucky

GUEST EDITOR

ROBIN DONOHOE DENNISON, DNP, APRN, CCNS, CEN, CNE
Associate Professor, Georgetown University, School of Nursing and Health Studies, Washington, DC

AUTHORS

MOLLIE E. ALESHIRE, DNP, FNP-BC, PNP-BC
Assistant Professor, College of Nursing, University of Kentucky, Lexington, Kentucky

DOROTHY BROOTEN, PhD, RN, FAAN
Professor of Nursing, Florida International University College of Nursing and Health Sciences, Miami, Florida

ANITA DEMPSEY, PhD, APRN, PMHCNS-BC
Assistant Professor of Nursing, Wright State University, College of Nursing and Health, Dayton, Ohio

ROBIN DONOHOE DENNISON, DNP, APRN, CCNS, CEN, CNE
Associate Professor, Georgetown University, School of Nursing and Health Studies, Washington, DC

DEBORA M. DOLE, PhD, CNM, RN
Faculty, College of Nursing, Academic Health Center, University of Cincinnati, Cincinnati, Ohio

JO ANN WALSH DOTSON, PhD, RN
Assistant Professor, College of Nursing, Washington State University, Spokane, Washington

DAWN DOUTRICH, PhD, RN, CNS
Associate Professor, College of Nursing, Washington State University, Vancouver, Washington

KATHLEEN FARRELL, DNSc, BC, CCNS, ARNP
Associate Professor, Murray State University, Murray, Kentucky

ANITA FINKELMAN, MSN, RN
Visiting Faculty, Bouvé College of Health Sciences, School of Nursing, Northeastern University, Boston, Massachusetts

KELLY A. GOUDREAU, DSN, RN, ACNS-BC
Past President, National Association of Clinical Nurse Specialists; Associate Director for Patient Care Services/Nurse Executive, Veterans Affairs Southern Oregon Rehabilitation Center and Clinics, White City, Oregon

FRANK GUIDO-SANZ, MSN, ARNP
PhD Candidate, Florida International University College of Nursing and Health Sciences, Miami, Florida

JEAN HANNAN, PhD, ARNP
Assistant Professor of Nursing, Florida International University College of Nursing and Health Sciences, Miami, Florida

MARTHE J. MOSELEY, PhD, RN, CCNS
Associate Director, Clinical Practice, Office of Nursing Service, Veterans Health Care Administration, Washington, DC; Professor of Nursing, Rocky Mountain University of Health Professions, Provo, Utah

CYNTHIA F. NYPAVER, MSN, CNM, WHNP-BC
Faculty and Doctoral Student, College of Nursing, Academic Health Center, University of Cincinnati, Cincinnati, Ohio

STEPHEN PATTEN, MSN, RN, CNS, CNOR
President, National Association of Clinical Nurse Specialists; Clinical Nurse Specialist, Operative Care Division, Veterans Affairs Portland Oregon Medical Center, Portland, Oregon

CAMILLE PAYNE, PhD, RN
Professor, Kennesaw State University, Kennesaw, Georgia

SUZANNE S. PREVOST, PhD, RN, COI
Associate Dean, Practice and Community Engagement, University of Kentucky, Lexington, Kentucky

JUDY RIBAK, PhD, APRN, PMHCNS-BC
Assistant Professor of Nursing, Wright State University, College of Nursing and Health, Dayton, Ohio

JOAN M. STANLEY, PhD, RN, CRNP, FAAN, FAANP
Senior Director of Education Policy, American Association of Colleges of Nursing, Washington, DC

TUKEA L. TALBERT, DNP, RN
Chief Nursing Officer, Clark Regional Medical Center, Winchester, Kentucky

KATHY WHEELER, PhD, FNP-BC, FAANP
Assistant Professor, College of Nursing, University of Kentucky, Lexington, Kentucky

WANDA O. WILSON, CRNA, PhD, MSN
Executive Director, American Association of Nurse Anesthetists, Park Ridge, Illinois

JOANNE M. YOUNGBLUT, PhD, RN, FAAN
Professor of Nursing, Florida International University College of Nursing and Health Sciences, Miami, Florida

Contents

a more efficient and effective health care system. Certified registered nurse anesthetists will help manage this change by continuing to provide patient access to safe, cost-effective anesthesia care; knowing the direction in which health care is headed; being politically active at the state and federal levels; educating the public about the value of nurse anesthetists; and being involved at the local community and institutional levels.

integration of advanced practice registered nurses (APRNs) into an organization. The critical areas that nurse executives must consider to foster and empower APRNs are: (1) knowledge and self preparation, especially of political initiatives that affect the role, (2) visionary leadership and development of clear role expectations and appropriate credentialing, (3) strategies to reduce disconnection between the APRN and their practice setting, and (4) appropriate education and marketing of the role to stakeholders.

The advanced practice registered nurse (APRN) is vital in role-modeling and ensuring evidence-based practice (EBP) engagement and application at the point of care. This article describes the formulation of national competencies for EBP, specific to the APRN level. The application of selected competencies is delineated and the creation of an APRN action plan to identify necessary EBP competencies is discussed. If EBP skills are lacking, the action plan is used for development of skills in the required areas.

Interprofessional collaboration was essential for the conduct of research that demonstrated the effectiveness and significance of advanced practice registered nurses (APRNs) in providing care, in reducing health care costs, and in developing innovative models of care for the nation's citizens. If the 2010 Affordable Care Act is to be implemented, APRNs, with their expertise and numbers, are essential to its implementation. Continued interdisciplinary collaboration is needed to expand the scope of APRN state practice regulations, to change reimbursement for APRN services, and to mute opposition to these changes by medical organizations.

The role of the psychiatric mental health clinical nurse specialist (PMHCNS) is now in a precarious position. At first glance, some may say it is on the verge of extinction. In this article, a brief history of the role of the PMHCNS is reviewed along with current education, practice, role, and American Nurses Credentialing Center certification of the PMHCNS. The future implications and considerations of the unique functions of the PMHCNS for an advanced practice registered nurse with a psychiatric mental health specialization are discussed.

This article addresses the need for continued certification of community and public health nurses at the advanced practice registered nurse level, and explores curricular avenues and policy recommendations with regard to certification and education of these nurses. The transformation of health care and burgeoning access to information has changed what the public expects and needs from health professionals. Nursing roles have expanded and transformed, in turn requiring that the education, licensure, certification, and accreditation of the professional likewise change.

NURSING CLINICS
OF NORTH AMERICA

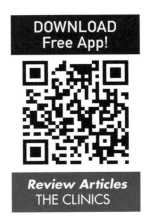

Preface

This is a dynamic time for advanced practice registered nurses (APRNs), fraught with both opportunities and challenges. In the recent *Institute of Medicine* publication *The Future of Nursing*, four key messages were emphasized.[1] First, "nurses should practice to the full extent of their education and training." This message is especially important to APRNs, who have advanced education and scope of practice but significant restrictions on their practice in many states. This IOM report recommended that scope-of-practice barriers be removed.

Second, the IOM recommends that "nurses should achieve higher levels of education and training through an education system that promotes seamless academic progression." Education for advanced practice has moved from certificate programs for registered nurses to master's degree programs and now a practice doctorate. The report recommends that the number of nurses with a doctorate be doubled by 2020. The addition of the option of a practice doctorate (ie, Doctor in Nursing Practice) to the previous option of a research doctorate (ie, Doctor of Philosophy) provides a new opportunity for nurses who are focused on nursing practice and practice leadership. The report also emphasizes that nurses be engaged in lifelong learning to remain current and gain additional competencies.

Third, the IOM report states that "nurses should be full partners in redesigning health care in the United States." The report emphasizes that nurses should be enabled to lead change and assume leadership positions in public, private, and governmental agencies. Finally, the report concludes that "effective workforce planning and policy making require better data collection and information infrastructure" to project workforce requirements.

This report and other changes in the landscape of advanced practice nursing can be viewed as either an opportunity or a threat. This issue begins with articles specifically describing the past, present, and future of each of the APRN roles: nurse midwife, nurse practitioner, nurse anesthetist, and clinical nurse specialist. These are followed by articles discussing crucial aspects of advanced practice nursing such as evidence-based practice and collaboration, as well as factors that will have a significant impact on advanced practice nursing such as the Consensus Model and the Doctorate in Nursing Practice. Also included are discussions on the role of the nurse executive in facilitating the role of the APRN and the implications of the IOM reports on the role of the APRN. Finally, there are discussions of some controversial changes in advanced practice within specific nursing specialties of psychiatric/mental health and public health.

Nurs Clin N Am 47 (2012) xi–xii
doi:10.1016/j.cnur.2012.04.004
0029-6465/12/$ – see front matter © 2012 Elsevier Inc. All rights reserved.

It is my hope that this issue will stimulate discussion about the future of APRN roles and how we can increase the influence of the work of these skilled professionals in the improvement of health care outcomes for all.

Robin Donohoe Dennison, DNP, APRN, CCNS, CEN, CNE
Georgetown University
School of Nursing and Health Studies
3700 Reservoir Road
Washington, DC 20057, USA

E-mail address:
rddennison@aol.com

REFERENCE

1. Institute of Medicine. The future of nursing: leading change, advancing health. 2010. Available at: http://www.iom.edu/Reports/2010/The-Future-of-Nursing-Leading-Change-Advancing-Health.aspx. Accessed March 30, 2012.

The Future of Nurse Practitioner Practice: A World of Opportunity

Mollie E. Aleshire, DNP, FNP-BC, PNP-BC[a],*,
Kathy Wheeler, PhD, FNP-BC[b], Suzanne S. Prevost, PhD, RN, COI[c]

KEYWORDS

- Nurse practitioner • Role • Future of health care • Outcomes • Nursing
- Advanced registered nurse practitioner • Advanced practice

KEY POINTS

- Recent regulatory and policy developments give NPs the opportunity to be facilitators of cost-effective care models that improve access and quality of care.
- In an evolving health care system, NPs can positively impact health care delivery by focusing on health promotion, health maintenance, and prevention.
- In acute and primary care settings, NPs have a pivotal role in meeting the health care needs of an expanding, aging, and chronically ill population.
- Around the world, the NP's role must continue to be developed and clarified to benefit health care systems and health care consumers.
- NPs must seize the current opportunity to advance the role of the NP and must collaborate to transform and improve health care globally.

Health care around the world is transforming at a rate and in ways never seen previously. Nurses should be leading change and advancing health in an increasingly complex health system, according to the United States' Institute of Medicine (IOM) 2011 report, *The Future of Nursing*. The IOM report indicates "advanced practice registered nurses (APRNs) should be able to practice to the full extent of their education and training."[1] This recommendation and the multiple systemic health care changes occurring secondary to the United States' 2010 Patient Protection and Affordable Care Act (PPACA) make this an optimal time for full use of nurse practitioners (NPs) in ways not realized previously. This article describes the evolution and future of the NP role,

The authors have nothing to disclose.
[a] College of Nursing, University of Kentucky, 450A CON Building, Lexington, KY 40536-0232, USA
[b] College of Nursing, University of Kentucky, 450C CON Building, Lexington, KY 40536-0232, USA
[c] Practice and Community Engagement, College of Nursing, University of Kentucky, 750 Rose Street, Lexington, KY 40536-0232, USA
* Corresponding author.
E-mail address: mollie.aleshire@uky.edu

explores the practice in relation to regulation and policy; primary care; acute care; international, global, and cultural issues; and public image, and addresses how NPs must prepare for changing health care environments and consumer demands.

The NP role was first conceptualized in the United States in 1965 when Loretta Ford and Henry Silver began a certificate program at the University of Colorado that provided nurses with the skills to provide primary care to children in the community. Soon, multiple certificate programs for NPs formed in an effort to fill gaps in the supply of physicians in rural areas. In the early years, the NP was defined as a nurse with advanced training and skills who had a responsibility for health care, using knowledge and skills from the disciplines of both nursing and medicine to provide primary care. In the 1970s, NP education began to move from certificate programs to bachelor's and master's degree programs. Although often still focusing on primary care, from the 1970s forward the NP role evolved to include adult/geriatrics, family, women's health, neonatal, acute care, and other specialty roles. Skills in leadership, affecting change, and decision making also became an integral expectation of the NP role, and NP certification became a common expectation.[2]

By the 1980s, more NPs began to provide services in acute care settings, and the elaboration of conceptual models of the role and diversification of NP roles proceeded. In the 1980s and 1990s, several NP organizations were formed to advance the NP profession. By the mid-1990s, NP was a broadly defined term generally referring to a health care provider with graduate-level preparation, certification, and the potential to practice in a variety of settings. Subsequently, descriptions of the role of the NP became more detailed but continued to differ widely among regions, settings, and organizations.[2] Also in the 1990s, graduate programs were established to specifically prepare nurses for the acute care NP (ACNP) role, and a certification unique to that role was offered for the first time in 1995.

A defining moment in NP practice evolution occurred when the Balanced Budget Act of 1997 granted NPs provider status and authorized them to bill Medicare directly for services. Multiple definitions and understandings of NP practice continue to abound, differing from state to state and organization to organization. All states recognize NPs as health care providers, but individual state regulations vary widely regarding issues such as prescribing, reimbursement for services, and autonomy of practice.[2]

Similar advanced practice roles have developed throughout much of the world. Nurse anesthetists and nurse midwives first appeared in Korea in the 1950s, and NPs appeared in the 1980s.[3] Also in that decade, several other countries started using nurses in a variety of advanced practice roles, recently providing regulatory and supportive frameworks.[4] New provider roles have begun to evolve worldwide, all with the potential to substantially and positively influence health care. To ensure this happens, stakeholders must understand the vision and provide optimal structure and support.

REGULATION AND POLICY

The next several decades of NP practice in the United States will be defined by four significant policy and regulation initiatives: the Consensus Model for APRN Regulation, the Doctor of Nursing Practice (DNP) movement, the PPACA, and the IOM Future of Nursing Report. The consuming regulatory mission for the next several years for advanced practice nurses in the United States will be the implementation of the Consensus Model for APRN Regulation: Licensure, Accreditation, Certification, and Education (Consensus Model),[5] This undertaking will be the culmination of a multiyear endeavor involving more than 70 nursing and health care organizations,[6] producing a mandate for individual states to uniformly approach licensure, accreditation, certification, and education.[7] The absence of regulatory consistency has long been recognized as a significant hindrance to practice and patient care.

The Consensus Model has set out to accomplish the following things:

1. Define APRN as the licensing and practice title for those educated and functioning in one of four roles: certified NP (CNP), certified nurse-midwife (CNM), certified registered nurse anesthetist (CRNA), or clinical nurse specialist (CNS).[5]
2. Require graduates to complete a nationally accredited graduate program, either degree-granting or postgraduate.[5]
3. Make APRN education broad-based but population-focused (family/individual across the lifespan, adult-gerontology, pediatrics, neonatal, women's health/gender-related or psychological/mental health), with appropriate clinical and didactic material, that must include three separate graduate-level courses in advanced physiology/pathophysiology, health assessment, and pharmacology. Graduates must be eligible to sit for national certification intended for state licensure.[5]
4. Require certification examinations to be given through nationally accredited certification bodies, with examinations specific to role and population.[5]
5. Require those licensed as APRNs to be prepared to assume full role responsibilities, including health promotion, health maintenance, assessment, diagnosis, and problem management, through both pharmacologic and nonpharmacologic means.[5]

When implementation of these recommendations is added to the DNP movement, it becomes clear that NPs, regulators, educators, administrators, and policy makers have not only great potential for progress but also a lot at stake in terms of NP licensing, accreditation, credentialing, and education. As leaders in each state refine their Nurse Practice Acts, NPs will need to be vigilant in participation and oversight to reach regulatory consistency.[6]

The PPACA, also referred to as the Affordable Care Act (ACA), although whittled down from its original broad intent to overhaul the US health care system, remains so sweeping in its potential that its full effect for APRNs is difficult to foresee. Now limited primarily to insurance reform, it provides the opportunity to transform advanced practice. Both the ACA and the IOM Future of Nursing Report grew out of the realization that the US health care system is struggling. Reports such as those by The Commonwealth Fund show that the US health care system consistently underperforms relative to other developed countries in terms of multiple parameters; is the most expensive in the world; and suffers from lack of nurse coordination for chronic illness.[8] NPs must be knowledgeable and prepared to attend to all of the recommendations and initiatives. The IOM[1] recommends the following: eliminate scope-of-practice barriers, increase collaborative improvement efforts, develop nurse residency programs, double the number of nurses with doctorate degrees, engage nurses in lifelong learning, and prepare nurses to be change agents for a better health care system. The ACA recommends new models of care to provide cost savings while improving health care delivery, such as through community health centers, medical homes, accountable care organizations, and insurance exchanges. These efforts provide great opportunity for NPs to contribute to increased access and quality of care, but only if they are actively participating.

Policy revisions are needed to control costs and improve health care through the more effective use of nurses. NPs, in particular, need to affect the economics of the prevention of disease and those of treatment. Prevention must be a priority. If prevention is successful, which is where the stream of cost begins, the expense of treating disease downstream can be lessened significantly. Patients and families are drowning in this river of costs, but through pulling them from the stream quickly, their expenses are lessened and critical resources of the health care system are preserved. If policymakers can determine how best to do this, money and lives can be saved. NPs must participate in creating these policies by promoting good health through disease and injury prevention, thereby winning at upstream health care economics. This effort includes improving the social determinants of health, such as balanced nutrition and safe housing.[9]

As populations age, and especially when upstream policies have not done a good job at preventing risk factors such as obesity and smoking, the health care system is facing overwhelming chronic disease. Treatment for these problems is resource-intensive. Nurses and NPs may be the best solution, not simply because of cost savings, but because of proven records of success and closeness to the patient. Perhaps it is time, as recommends Dr Tesfamicael Ghebrehiwet[10] of the International Council of Nurses, for them to be the health care providers known for managing the noncommunicable diseases facing the world.

These significant health care issues all require strong policy initiatives and the political will to make them happen; however, the issue is much broader than the profession of nursing and advanced practice nursing alone. NPs and related stakeholders must realize that this is an opportunity the nursing profession and US health care system really cannot afford to let slip away.

PRIMARY CARE

Evidence strongly suggests that the demand for primary care services in the United States will continue to exceed the supply of these services.[11] The US population is increasing, and within this decade baby boomers will begin to be eligible for Medicare. By 2030, one-fifth of Americans will be older than 65 years.[12] By 2025, the population growth and increased proportion of elderly individuals is expected to increase the number of ambulatory care visits by 29%.[13] Additionally, the percentage of the US population with chronic medical conditions is increasing. Currently, 45% of the US population have one chronic illness and approximately half of these have multiple chronic issues.[12,14,15]

If the ACA is sustained, it will increase the number of Americans with health care coverage, adding a projected 32 million individuals and expanding the percentage of US citizens with coverage from 83% to 94%. The ACA does this in the following ways:

1. By mandating that everyone obtain health care coverage or pay a fine
2. By developing high-risk insurance pools for those with health conditions that make it difficult to acquire affordable individually purchased coverage
3. By developing state-based health insurance exchanges through which small businesses and uninsured individuals can purchase health insurance
4. By reforming health insurance (eliminating maximum lifetime limits, eliminating denial for preexisting conditions, eliminating coverage cancellation due to illness, eliminating higher premiums due to preexisting conditions, and allowing coverage of dependents until 26 years of age)
5. By expanding Medicaid coverage to all people younger than 65 years in households with incomes up to 138% of the federal poverty level.[16]

Despite the increasing demand for primary care, the number of primary care physicians is decreasing. Many primary care physicians are retiring or leaving primary care, and the number of US medical school graduates entering general internal medicine or family practice residencies continues to decline.[17–20] A shortage of 35,000 to 44,000 primary care physicians is projected to occur in the United States by 2024.[13] In contrast, the number of nurses entering and graduating from primary care NP programs continues to increase.[21]

The United States has the most expensive health care system in the world, spending far more per capita on health care than other developed countries. The per capita spending is nearly double the average for developed countries in the world, and the United States continues to increase its health care spending at a faster rate than other similar wealthy countries. Despite this high cost, the US health care system does not achieve better outcomes than other countries,[22] and underperforms relative to other countries on measures such as quality, access, efficiency, equity, morbidity, and mortality.[23] Many other developed countries have health care systems that more fully use primary care services and place a much higher emphasis on health promotion and prevention strategies. In other countries, the concept of the "medical home" has been more fully realized, with patients reporting having a primary care provider and receiving primary care services more consistently. This emphasis on primary care has been shown to account for a significant portion of the improved health outcomes seen in other countries.[23]

NPs provide quality care in a cost-effective manner. When patient outcomes of care managed by NPs are compared with care managed exclusively by physicians, the outcomes are comparable and in some instances better.[24–29] NP care and physician care have shown at least equivalent patient outcomes in areas such as glucose control,[24,26] hemoglobin A1C control,[24,26] patient satisfaction,[25,26,28,30] self-reported patient perception of health,[25,26] asthma control,[26] blood pressure control,[26] functional status,[25] lipid control,[25] emergency department or urgent care visits,[25] rates of hospitalization,[25] readmission rates,[27] hospital length of stay,[25,27] and mortality rates.[25,27] Additionally, lower costs are associated with NP care. The average cost of an NP primary care office visit is approximately 25% to 30% less than the average physician primary care office visit.[21]

Increased use of NPs is one of the most cost-effective and feasible ways to help meet the need for health care in the United States that is of high quality, accessible, and affordable.[31] As health care continues to rapidly evolve in the coming decade, expansion in patient-centered medical homes, NP-led clinics, and convenient care clinics is anticipated.[32,33] NPs will be health care providers in each of these care delivery models.[23,33,34] A new focus on primary care, health promotion, and prevention has become essential, and NPs have historically provided care in a model focused on prevention.

ACUTE CARE

As the demand for primary care services is growing, a simultaneous growth in demand for acute care providers is occurring. ACNPs, with specialty education at the graduate level, are well prepared to respond to several needs in acute care settings and in some specialty clinics that provide care to patients with high-acuity illnesses, such as cardiology practices. Just as the primary care NP role originally evolved in response to a physician shortage, recently imposed limitations on medical resident work hours (no more than 16 consecutive hours and no more than 80 hours per week) have created an urgent need for more providers with specialty expertise to manage the care of patients in acute care settings on a 24-hour basis.[35] The need is particularly critical in academic medical centers that have historically relied on medical residents for around-the-clock coverage of acute and critically ill patients. Many of these institutions are actively recruiting ACNPs to fill this void, and the demand is projected to increase.[35]

ACNPs are also contributing to enhanced quality of care and cost-effectiveness in acute care settings. Many ACNPs lead interprofessional teams focused on enhancing and documenting clinical quality improvement initiatives, such as the core measures documentation required by the Joint Commission, or the measurement and documentation of nursing-sensitive indicators required for magnet hospital designation. Additionally, ACNPs respond to patients experiencing acute physical deterioration by staffing rapid response teams in hospitals.[36] Consistent with the historical NP emphasis on preventive care, ACNPs focus much of their work on the prevention of iatrogenic complications and illnesses.

The NP role emphasizes health promotion, health maintenance, prevention, and detection of alterations in health through supportive interventions, counseling, and teaching of families, staff, and other providers. The role includes illness care management, such as diagnosis and management of common, chronic, and acute conditions. NP practice is based on an epidemiologic approach to health problems, an understanding of community and institutional systems, the management of resources, and the use of appropriate technology. NP's roles in both primary and acute care will continue to evolve and grow. Because of their preparation and model of care, NPs will have a pivotal position in health care, responding to the demographic and epidemiologic demands of an expanding, aging, and chronically ill population.[37]

INTERNATIONAL, GLOBAL, AND CULTURAL ISSUES

As the world has become more mobile and communities more diverse, the opportunities and responsibilities for NPs have broadened. Countries outside the United States have embraced the NP role and are working through the licensing, accreditation, credentialing, and educational issues inherent to effective role development, often with assistance from NPs in the United States. NPs organize and participate in medical brigades throughout the world. Along with nurses, NPs are involved in helping to achieve the United Nations' Millennium Development Goals. Schools of nursing build curriculums to educate and attend to cultural issues and health literacy, aware that students need this material for patients in the United States and any experiences the students might have outside the United States. These endeavors will accelerate and expand, and nurses in and out of the United States will need to be informed, thoughtful, and collaborative to achieve optimal outcomes. As these opportunities arise, encouraging self-determinism rather than dictating the process will be particularly important, and can best be accomplished through modeling best practices, sharing supportive documents, including historical explanations, with an intentional emphasis on cultural sensitivity and cultural appropriateness. As NPs and other nurses engage in international collaboration, all partners will need to respect the reciprocal value of the learning process.

The NP role is rapidly emerging worldwide. A 2004 survey of International Nurse Practitioner/Advanced Practice Nursing Network (INP/APNN) members found that 60 countries had or were in the process of developing the field of advanced practice nursing in some form.[38] A similar survey performed in 2008 found 13 different titles represented the role; 71% of the countries had NP education within the country, and a master's degree was the level of education 50% of the time.[39] This finding represents significant progress and is cause for celebration. However, the lack of consistency has made it difficult to interpret outcomes or plan research.[40] This must be noted in light of similar, though milder problems of consistency in the United States, hence the need for the Consensus Model to standardize advanced practice in the United States.

As a young profession, the structures to support these many efforts are in their formative stages. Three US organizations attend specifically to NP issues. In 2000, the International Council of Nurses (ICN) and the American Academy of Nurse Practitioners (AANP) jointly created the INP/APNN, intended to assist NPs in role development throughout the world.[41,42] Aside from customary networking and communication services, the INP/APNN sponsors periodic international conferences that are well attended and growing. The second and third NP organizations involved in international issues are the AANP and National Organization of Nurse Practitioner Faculties, which have both created standing subcommittees devoted exclusively to international interests. None of the three organizations participate in coordinating or providing direct care to patients in these settings. However, through communication networks and the research and publications of these organizations, sufficient materials have been created to illuminate the NP role in the United States. One particularly helpful document is the 2008 ICN publication *Scope of Practice, Standards and Competencies of the Advanced Practice Nurse*, addressing practice and education.[42] With the 2002 decision of the ICN to recommend a master's degree for entry into advanced practice,[4] the recent American Academy of Colleges of Nursing (AACN) publication of *The Essentials of Master's Education in Nursing*[43] may also be helpful. The document recommends that the core curriculum for APRN education be consistent with the Consensus Model.

Although the NP role has representation throughout the world, pronounced barriers limit the flow of nurses and advanced practice nurses across borders, whether to provide care or to seek education. According to Schober,[40] the issue is seen primarily in three areas: NPs in other countries hoping to practice in the United States, nurses from other countries who enter US NP programs hoping to return home to function as NPs, and nurses outside the United States hoping to enter NP programs in the United States. Despite the efforts of the Commission on Graduates of Foreign Nursing Schools, the problem of nurses outside the United States wishing to enter US programs remains the most burdensome. For practitioners to have the fluidity needed to meet global needs in terms of direct care and education, especially during times of crisis, some resolution is needed. The same is true in terms of the need for accreditation or credentialing of NP education programs throughout the world. It may be time to lay the groundwork for that, just as medical schools have done. The World Federation for Medical Education performs this function for medical schools. Currently this is voluntary, but recommendations have been made for the system to become mandatory.[44] In all likelihood, NPs and NP education programs are on the same path, or should be.

PUBLIC IMAGE

Despite being comparatively new, the NP profession celebrated its 45th birthday during the summer of 2010. Forty-five years should be sufficient time for a profession to define itself in the eyes of the public. However, a 2010 media study by the AANP found that the public continues to be confused about the role, education, abilities, and success of NPs, with many not knowing NPs order tests or prescribe medications.[45] Although continuously voted the most trusted profession,[46] nursing has struggled to fully define itself to the public. Finding that only 4% of health care articles made any reference to nursing, the Woodhull Study on Nursing and the Media stated, "Nurses and the nursing profession are essentially invisible to the media and, consequently, to the American public."[47]

Even major marketing campaigns, such as The Nurse Practitioner National Marketing Campaign,[48] operational from 2000 to 2003, and Johnson & Johnson's

Campaign for Nursing's Future,[49] operational since 2002, have not fully succeeded in defining nursing or advanced practice nursing to the public. Certainly the confusion of nursing titles has compounded the problem. Adding the title of DNP may increase the confusion, at least in the short term, unless countermeasures are well planned. Some have suggested that the dialogue over title use for NPs and DNPs should be minimized so that the public only hears the words *nurse, physician,* and *nurse practitioner*.[50] Others feel that earning a doctorate, with all of the earned privileges, such as use of title, is one of the best ways to improve the image of NPs.

Regardless of how this debate concludes, the public likes and trusts NPs and sees them as a solution to limited access to care. After 4 decades of providing care to patients, the public is beginning to understand the term *nurse practitioner* and understand some level of function. The 2010 AANP media study found that 81% of Americans have seen an NP themselves or know someone significant to them who has. This finding shows the extent of reach of NP and reflects title recognition and a beginning understanding of the role. These consumers also believed that NPs improved and expedited access to care and spent more time listening to patient concerns than other providers.[45]

With these issues in mind, NPs have been taking on the task of better defining the role by attempting to harness the power of the media. Nurses and NPs are starting to host radio shows, such as Partners in Practice by NP Mimi Secor[51] and Healthstyles by Diana Mason and Barbara Glickstein.[52] It is important for NPs to continue to publicize the mantra of providing patient-centered, accessible, affordable, quality care. This message has been framed for NPs, and now it is time for broad dissemination by effectively using public media. Whenever possible, NPs must affect their image via traditional media such as newspapers, radio, and television, but also via social media such as blogs, Facebook, Twitter, and YouTube.[53] To assist with that process, the AANP and others have offered media training. NPs need to take advantage of this training, recognizing that every encounter with a patient, pharmacist, physician, coworker, or administrator is an opportunity to affect image. NPs should create a personal media package, including not only a quick elevator message of what an NP is but also a variety of marketing materials, such as professional cards, informative pamphlets about NPs, and patient educational materials containing NP name, credentials, and practice information. When working with social media such as Facebook and MySpace, NPs must be cognizant of the image issues of the NP and the organizations they may be viewed as representing. They must be careful about "friending" patients or sharing patient information that violates the Health Insurance Portability and Accountability Act (HIPAA). Because of concerns regarding these issues, the American Nurses Association has recently published Principles for Social Networking and the Nurse, assisting nurses to understand the issues and how to avoid problems.[54]

Significant positive image effects can be expected from work flowing from the IOM Future of Nursing and the related action coalitions, which are charged with overseeing implementation of significant recommendations at all levels of nursing. NPs must participate as fully as possible in all of these endeavors, assisting the action coalitions and getting the NP message out, thereby meeting the goal of improved access to patient-centered, affordable, accessible quality health care.

A WORLD OF OPPORTUNITY

The foundation has been built and it is up to stakeholders to advance the role of the NP, to capitalize on the investment, and empower the movement. As Fairman and colleagues[55] recently stated, "fighting the expansion of NPs' scope of practice is no longer a defensible strategy. The challenge will be for all health care professionals to embrace these changes and come together to improve US health care." Because the world's health is at stake, the largest group of health care providers, nurses, must lead the effort in quality, coordination, and efficiency in a dynamic health care system. NPs have a phenomenal opportunity to collaborate with other health care professionals to improve community and global health.[34]

With so many opportunities open to NPs, the path must include engagement in educational preparation, research, role advocacy, interprofessional collaboration, leadership, patient advocacy, and system coordination. For the coming decades, NPs will need additional skills in leadership, business, economics, health policy, media, and technology. At the same time, NPs must continue to provide quality, patient-centered, cost-effective, evidence-based care.

Discussion of regulation and policy, primary care, acute care, NP education, global issues, and public image shows the indispensable and evolving role of the NP. The opportunity to leverage the wonderful care provided by NPs and other APRNs to transform health care should not be underestimated. The future is very bright for NPs and the nursing profession.

REFERENCES

1. Institute of Medicine (IOM). The future of nursing: leading change, advancing health. Washington, DC: The National Academies Press; 2011.
2. Sullivan-Marx E, McGivern D, Fairman J, et al, editors. Nurse Practitioners: the evolution and future of advanced practice. 5th edition. New York: Springer Publishing Company; 2010.
3. Kim D. The APN in Korea. Presented at the International Conference of Nurses Conference. Geneva, June 27, 2003.
4. Schober M, Affara F. Advanced nursing practice. Malden (MA): Blackwell Publishing; 2006.
5. Consensus model for APRN regulation: licensure, accreditation, certification & education. 2008. Available at: http://www.aacn.nche.edu. Accessed August 15, 2011.
6. O'Grady ET, Ford LC. The politics of advanced practice nursing. In: Mason DJ, Leavitt JK, Chafee MW, editors. Policy & politics in nursing and health care. St Louis (MO): Elsevier; 2012. p. 393–400.
7. Stanley J. Reaching consensus on a regulatory model: what does this mean for APRNs? J Nurse Pract 2009;11(4):8–23.
8. Davis K, Schoen C, Schoenbaum SC, et al. Mirror, mirror on the wall: an international update on the comparative performance of American health care. New York: The Commonwealth Fund; 2007.
9. Kawachi I. Paddling upstream: contributions of social determinants to population health. Paper presented at: BlueCross and BlueShield of Minnesota Foundation Statewide Policy Forum on Social Determinants of Health. Eagan, November 13, 2006.
10. Ghebrehiwet T. International health and policy: WHA and nursing resolutions. The what, why and how? Paper presented at: International Council of Nurses Global Nursing Leadership Institute. Geneva, September 10, 2011.
11. American College of Physicians. How is a shortage of primary care physicians affecting the quality and cost of medical care? Philadephia: American College of Physicians; 2008.
12. Wu S, Green A. Projection of chronic illness prevalence and cost inflation. Santa Monica (CA): RAND Health; 2000.

13. Colwill JM, Cultice JM, Kruse RL. Will generalist physician supply meet demands of an increasing and aging population? Health Aff 2008;27(3):w232–41.
14. Anderson GF. Medicare and chronic conditions. N Engl J Med 2005;353(3):305–9.
15. Hoffman C, Schwartz K. Eroding access among nonelderly U.S. adults with chronic conditions: Ten years of change. Health Aff 2008;27(5):w340–8.
16. Keehan SP, Sisko AM, Truffer CJ, et al. National health spending projections through 2020: economi recovery and reform drive faster spending growth. Health Aff 2011;30(8):1594–605.
17. American Academy of Pediatrics Committee on Pediatric Workforce. Pediatrician workforce statement. Pediatrics 2005;116(1):263–9.
18. Hauer KE, Alper EJ, Clayton CP, et al. Educational responses to declining student interest in internal medicine careers. Am J Med 2005;118(10):1164–70.
19. Lipner RS, Bylsma WH, Arnold GK, et al. Who is maintaining certification in internal medicine–and why? A national survey 10 years after initial certification. Ann Intern Med 2006;144(1):29–36.
20. Pugno PA, McGaha AL, Schmittling GT, et al. Results of the 2007 National Resident Matching Program: family medicine. Fam Med 2007;39(8):562–71.
21. Naylor MD, Kurtzman ET. The role of nurse practitioners in reinventing primary care. Health Aff 2010;39(5):893–9.
22. The Henry J. Kaiser Family Foundation. Health care spending in the United States and selected OECD countries. April 2011. Available at: http://www.kff.org/insurance/snapshot/OECD042111.cfm. Accessed October 9, 2011.
23. Davis K, Schoen C, Stremikis K. Mirror, mirror on the wall: how the performance of the U.S. health care system compares internationally—2010 update. New York: The Commonwealth Fund; 2010.
24. Conlon P. Diabetes outcomes in primary care: evaluation of the diabetes nurse practitioner compared to the physician. Prim Health Care 2010;20(5):26–31.
25. Newhouse RP, Stanik-Hutt J, White KM, et al. Advanced practice nurse outcomes 1990-2008: a systematic review. Nurs Econ 2011;29(5):230–50.
26. Mundinger M, Kane R, Lenz E, et al. Primary care outcomes in patients treated by nurse practitioners or physicians. JAMA 2000;283(1):59–68.
27. Hoffman L, Tasota F, Zullo T, et al. Outcomes of care managed by an acute care nurse practitioner/attending physician team in a subacute medical intensive care unit. Am J Crit Care 2005;14(2):121–32.
28. Guzik A, Menzel N, Fitzpatrick J, et al. Patient satisfaction with nurse practitioner and physician services in the occupational health setting. AAOHN J 2009;57(5):191–7.
29. Chen C, McNeese-Smith D, Cowan M, et al. Evaluation of a nurse practitioner-led care management model in reducing inpatient drug utilization and cost. Nurs Econ 2009;27(3):160–8.
30. Deirick-van Daele A, Metsemakers J, Derckx E, et al. Nurse practitioners substituting for general practitioners: randomized controlled trial. J Adv Nurs 2009;65(2):391–401.
31. Bauer J. Nurse practitioners as an underutilized resource for health reform: evidence-based demonstrations of cost-effectiveness. J Am Acad Nurse Pract 2010;22(4):228–31.
32. Tobler L. A primary problem. State Legis 2010;20–4.
33. Miller K. Consumer-driven health care: nurse practitioners making history. J Nurse Pract 2009;5(1):31–4.
34. Koeniger-Donohue R, Hawkins J. The future of nursing and health care: through the looking glass 2030. J Am Acad Nurse Pract 2010;22:233–5.

35. Pastores SM, O'Connor MF, Kleinpell RM, et al. The Accreditation Council for Graduate Medical Education resident duty hour new standards: history, changes, and impact on staffing of intensive care units. Crit Care Med 2011;39(11):2540–9.
36. Landsperger JS, Williams KJ, Hellervik SM, et al. Implementation of a medical intensive care unit acute-care nurse practitioner service. Hosp Pract (Minneap) 2011;39(2):32–9.
37. Ford LC. Celebrate the past and create a vision for the future. J Am Acad Nurse Pract 2010;22:177.
38. Roodbol P. INP/APNN 2004 conference survey. Gronigan (The Netherlands): INP/APNN; 2004.
39. Pulcini J, Jelic M, Gul R, et al. An international survey on advanced practice nursing education, practice, and regulation. J Nurs Scholarsh 2010;42(1):31–9.
40. Schober M. International report to AANP board of directors. Washington, DC: American Academy of Nurse Practitioners; 2011.
41. International Council of Nurses. ICN Nurse Practitioner/Advanced Practice Network. Available at: http://www.icn-apnetwork.org/. Accessed August 15, 2011.
42. ICN International Nurse Practitioner/Advanced Practice Nursing Network. Scope of practice, standards and competencies of the advanced practice nurse. Geneva (Switzerland): International Council of Nurses; 2008.
43. American Association of Colleges of Nursing. The essentials of master's education in nursing. Available at: http://www.aacn.nche.edu/education-resources/MastersEssentials11.pdf. Accessed September 3, 2011.
44. Canadian Medical Association. Administrator calls for global health credentialing. Can Med Assoc J 2009;180(8):E11–2.
45. AANP/AANPF. The nurse practitioners media omnibus memo. Austin (TX): American Academy of Nurse Practitioners; 2010.
46. Nurses shine, bankers slump in ethics ratings. Gallup Web site. Available at: http://www.gallup.com/poll/112264/nurses-shine-while-bankers-slump-ethics-ratings.aspx. Accessed April 17, 2012.
47. Tau ST. The Woodhull study on nursing and the media: Health care's invisible partner. Indianapolis (IN): Center Nursing Press; 1997.
48. NP national marketing campaign. NP Central Web site. Available at: http://www.npcentral.net/mc/. Accessed August 15, 2011.
49. Preparing nurses for the future. Johnson & Johnson Web site. Available at: http://www.jnj.com/connect/caring/patient-stories/preparing-nurses-for-the-future. Accessed September 3, 2011.
50. Mills C. Defining nurse practitioners. Nurse Practitioner World News 2010;15(1/2):3.
51. Mimi Secor: nurse practitioner, speaker, consultant. Available at: http://mimisecor.com. Accessed September 3, 2011.
52. Healthstyles—Diana Mason, Barbara Glickstein. WBAI.org Web site. Available at: http://www.wbai.org/index.php?option=content&task=view&id=384&Itemid=42. Accessed September 3, 2011.
53. Mason D. Media, policy, and politics. Paper presented at: International Council of Nurses Global Nursing Leadership Institute. Geneva, September 10, 2011.
54. American Nurses Association. Principles for social networking and the nurse: guidelines for registered nurses. Silver Spring (MD): American Nurses Association; 2011.
55. Fairman JA, Rowe JW, Hassmiller S, et al. Broadening the scope of nursing practice. N Engl J Med 2011;364(3):193–6.

The Bright Future for Clinical Nurse Specialist Practice

Stephen Patten, MSN, RN, CNS, CNOR[a,*],
Kelly A. Goudreau, DSN, RN, ACNS-BC[b]

KEYWORDS

- CNS • Specialist • Expert • Future • Consensus
- Advanced practice registered nurse

KEY POINTS

- The perfect storm is here: health care reform, the Institute of Medicine's report, and the consensus model have all come together at one time. These 3 opportunities, along with the proliferation of institutions seeking magnet status, place the demand for the Clinical Nurse Specialists' (CNS) role at an all-time high.
- The CNS is trained to lead change in 3 of the most impactful areas of health care: direct patient care, nursing practice, and systems.
- Over the next several years, the demand for the work of CNS will grow exponentially, which will place a strain on the already-burdened nursing education system.

The future is full of opportunity and optimism for the Clinical Nurse Specialist (CNS) practice. It is a unique time in nursing history that carries tremendous importance, especially for CNSs. At present, there is a perfect storm of events that are culminating in a change in how health care will be delivered in the future in the United States. Health care reform is a work in progress and how it will ultimately look is unknown, but much of what is predicted holds promise for the continued growth of the CNS role.

As part of health care reform, the Patient Protection and Affordable Care Act, Public Law 111–148 (ACA),[1] is moving forward. What health care organizations described as the future in the ACA as accountable care organizations presents a great opportunity for CNSs with expectations of improved quality, safety, and assessment of health care outcomes for every American. The Institute of Medicine's (IOM) report on the Future of Nursing,[2] another major document released in the last 2 years, is nothing if not a call for CNSs to practice to the full extent of their training and education. CNSs are

[a] Operative Care Division, VA Portland Oregon Medical Center, 3710 Southwest US Veterans Hospital Road, Portland, OR 97239, USA
[b] VA Southern Oregon Rehabilitation Center and Clinics, 8495 Crater Lake Highway, White City, OR 97503, USA
* Corresponding author.
E-mail address: Stephen.Patten@va.gov

Nurs Clin N Am 47 (2012) 193–203
doi:10.1016/j.cnur.2012.02.009
0029-6465/12/$ – see front matter Published by Elsevier Inc.

nursing.theclinics.com

specifically educated to impact system change and improve the outcomes of nursing practice, which is a key concept in the report. Simultaneously, in an effort to retain high-quality care and the best nurses, many medical centers and hospitals have undertaken the journey to obtain Magnet status. The CNS has been documented in the literature to be in the perfect position to advance organizations in their Magnet journey.[3] Lastly but certainly not least is the Consensus Model for Advanced Practice Registered Nurses (APRN).[4] This new blueprint for all APRNs is widely accepted as the future for how licensure, accreditation, certification, and education will be accomplished in the future. All of these factors have now come together to give the CNS encouragement that the future is growing and improving.

Our future is bright. It is also built on the foundations of the past and the present. As we move to the future, we must understand the issues of the past and present to build on them to achieve what may be. Let this discussion of the past, the present, and the vision of the future guide decisions of CNS leaders in the future.

THE PAST

The role of the CNS presents a unique combination: a CNS is a nurse who is an expert nurse clinician who functions within a nursing specialty. This APRN operates in 3 distinct yet overlapping spheres of influence.[5] Within these spheres, the patient, nurse/nursing practice, and systems, the CNS uses evidence to develop or improve nursing practice, thus, improving patient outcomes. The foundations of the role are firmly centered in the essence of nursing practice and clinical expertise. Truly, the beginnings of this role reach as far back as Florence Nightingale's work during the Crimean War.[6] Nightingale, as an expert nurse clinician, worked within a specialty (trauma/combat) and used evidence to improve patient outcomes.

A new nursing role is only developed when there is a real or perceived need by society, the nursing profession, or the larger health care system. The role of the CNS grew from the societal and professional need for an expert clinician to guide peer nurses in areas of complex patient care and the reality that specialization was happening within health care and nursing.[7,8] The 2 separate phenomena, the need for an expert clinician and specialization, were developing simultaneously but actually developed independently of each other.[9] Hildegard Peplau brought the concepts together when she fully developed the psychiatric mental health CNS. The role further matured with the development of specialty competencies and role-specific competencies.[10] Evidence of societal and professional acceptance came over time: structured educational preparation that was CNS specific, educational programs became accredited, certification of individual CNSs was possible, and title protection/licensure occurred in some states.

The CNS role has been established as evidenced by discussions in the literature over the last 100 years. In a 1943 speech, Frances Reiter[7] talked about the "nurse clinician" as an expert nurse. She continued to refine her definition of this role for the next 40 years.[7] By 1966, she described the role as one with direct clinical practice and other indirect practices, such as activities carried out with other nurses and with other professionals but always on behalf of the patient.[7] This concept was identified as one of the conceptual beginnings of the 3 spheres of influence later described in the Statement on Clinical Nurse Specialist Practice and Education.[11] Reiter went on to further define this role as one that has a wide range of functions, an increased depth of understanding, and a provider of a wide breadth of services. The role of the expert clinician was seen as a part of nursing practice and as such needed to be controlled by nursing.[7] Not just any nurse could fill this role. The expert nurse clinician required experience, training, and a graduate-level education.[12]

Even before the discussion for the need of an expert nurse clinician, the need to specialize within nursing was being discussed. An *American Journal of Nursing* classic reprint of an October 1900 article by Katherine De Witt[13] describes a specialized nurse's sphere being more limited but patients getting better care now than when a nurse had to know and do it all. Dolores Little[8] expressed that specialization was no longer up for debate. She went on to describe a nurse specialist as one with advanced knowledge and skills in nursing practice regarding patients who have similar diseases, conditions, situations, or problems.[8]

In 1954, the 2 concepts of specialization and expert nursing care came together when Hildegard Peplau created a masters-level educational program for the preparation of psychiatric mental health clinical specialists at Rutgers.[14] By 1963, federal funding agencies were funding nurses to be trained as CNSs in a variety of specialties.[10] Although the role was fully established, there still existed some confusion. There were many different titles for CNSs with conflicting descriptions and unclear expectations of practice. In 1980, the American Nurses Association made clear their position with the release of their position statement, Nursing: A Social Policy Statement.[15] The statement clearly identified that the CNS must be educated at the graduate (masters or doctoral) level. It referred to specialization and expert practice as well as specialty certification. Most of the pieces were now in place to have the CNS role widely accepted in nursing, health care, and by society as a whole.

The National Association of Clinical Nurse Specialists (NACNS) was formed in 1995, and by 1996 the board of directors appointed an expert panel to develop core CNS competencies. After a rigorous multiple-tier process, including a review of the document by 51 nationally recognized nursing leaders and 9 national nursing organizations, the first Statement on Clinical Nurse Specialist Practice and Education was released in 1998.[16] The document contained the first set of fully described core CNS competencies and educational standards to be used in academe. The core competencies for all CNSs, regardless of specialty, were widely distributed and accepted. The final, and most recent, piece of the puzzle for recognition of the role was the creation of the Consensus Model for APRN Regulation: Licensure, Accreditation, Certification and Education.[4] This model was crafted to specifically spell out the requirements of the 4 roles of APRN: nurse practitioner, nurse midwife, nurse anesthetist, and the CNS. This process included more than 60 different organizations and took 4 years to complete. The document was widely accepted, and action is currently in process to fully implement the proposed regulatory model. Included in the model are title protection and recognition of CNSs as a full APRN role. This final piece has firmly established the role of the CNS in society and completed the process that started more than 100 years ago.

The CNS role, as with many other roles within nursing, had a colorful past that has taken many different turns along the way. The role is now well defined with core competencies that have gone through a third revision. Additional work undertaken by the NACNS includes a further-refined and updated list of specific education criteria that has been published in 2012. The NACNS is an organization that represents all CNSs regardless of specialty and is the steward of the CNS core competencies and the education criteria. The consensus model for APRN regulation has defined the requirements for licensure, accreditation, certification and education. All of the requirements to have a role accepted by nursing, health care, and society have now been met.

THE PRESENT

The world of the CNS has been changing rapidly over the past few years. The discussions of whether or not a CNS is an advanced practice nurse[17] and whether or not there were defined competencies[5] that had been clearly validated by the full spectrum of CNS practice and education have all been resolved in the last 3 years.[4,18,19] The additional changes that will be implemented by the acceptance and integration of the consensus model for APRN regulation will create challenges to the future. Current practice, however, continues to flow in a variety of areas.

The current practice for most CNSs continues to be in an acute care hospital setting, with some reaching out to the community and to specific populations of patients for specialty care and services. As clinical experts within the hospital setting, the CNS provides ongoing support to the care of complex patients, nursing and associated health staff, and the overall system of care.[5] These 3 spheres of influence provide an extraordinary framework for the full implementation of the various elements of the role. The elements include designing and evaluating nursing interventions, promoting innovation, change and diffusion of change across all practice areas, delivering care to complex clients, provision of consultation to other health care providers, mentoring the next generation of nurses, and addressing issues of integration of technology in the care environment.[19]

An area of great concern is that the practice of a CNS varies widely from state to state and even between health care organizations within the same state. CNSs can function as a clinical expert in a narrow specialty (ie, liver transplant) or a broad environment, such as medical/surgical nursing or community health. The depth of expertise varies depending on the needs of the environment.

The manner in which each CNS enacts their role is also variable. Some CNSs function within a specific population, such as adults or geriatric patient populations, and others function in a broad, across-the-lifespan environment, such as the emergency department or community health. This variability creates confusion and can lead to a misunderstanding or misinterpretation of the role by those who must understand it fully: the nursing staff, the nursing administrators, and the CNSs themselves. If the CNS cannot clearly articulate his or her role to the key stakeholders of nursing, then there is little hope that they can clearly define their value to those who enact the laws that impact the practice of CNSs in every state.

So what does the current practice of a CNS look like in its core elements regardless of the practice environment or the specialty that is the focus of the care provided? According to the National CNS Competency Task Force convened by NACNS to determine the core competencies for the CNS role, there are 7 core competencies defined with subelements that describe them fully to the level of implementation. The 7 core competencies are (1) direct care; (2) consultation; (3) systems leadership; (4) collaboration; (5) coaching; (6) research in the form of interpretation, translation and use of evidence, evaluation of clinical practice, and conduct of research; and (7) ethical decision making, moral agency, and advocacy.[18] These 7 core competencies are aligned within the 3 spheres of influence as described by the NACNS.[5]

The American Nurses Credentialing Center conducted a logical job analysis for the CNS core examination[20] that was intended to examine the core competencies of the CNS for the development of a core certification examination. They defined the core elements of CNS practice as the following: (1) phenomena of concern (ie, cognitive impairment, iatrogenesis, end of life, impaired wound healing, nausea, and so forth); (2) design and implementation of evidence-based nursing assessments, interventions, and programs with patients, families, communities, organizations, populations, or systems; (3) technology and the integration of products and devices; (4) teaching and coaching; (5) systems/organizations; (6) influencing change; (7) leadership, interdisciplinary collaboration, professionalism, and advocacy; (8) consultation; (9) measurement and evaluation; and (10) evidence-based practice and research.

Although similar, other than the semantics used to describe the concepts, these core elements of CNS practice are consistent with the core competencies identified by the NACNS CNS Competency Task Force.

Lewandowski and Adamle[21] described a comprehensive review of the literature regarding CNS practice. They identified more than 1200 articles representing CNS practice. These articles included anecdotal articles, research articles, dissertations and theses, abstracts, and presentations. Within this body of literature, they found 3 clear themes for the clinical practice of the CNS: management of the care of complex and vulnerable populations, education and support of interdisciplinary staff, and facilitation of change and innovation in health care systems.

The descriptions of CNS practice in Canada mirror these findings and go a little further because the role of the CNS in Canada has not been strictly defined by having a master's level of preparation. A recent study by Bryant-Lukosious (Bryant-Lukosious, personal communication, September 29, 2011) identified that CNSs in Canada fall into 2 distinct levels of education because a master's degree was not declared as the entry to practice for CNSs until 2008. Additionally, there is continued confusion in the role because of the low numbers in the work environment and some blending of the role to meet the needs of the clinical area that is being served. Bryant-Lukosious[22] identified that there is a clear distinction in the reported focal areas of the CNSs with and without a master's level of preparation. Those who were prepared at the master's level were able to articulate a level of nursing care that was more complex than the diploma- or baccalaureate-prepared nurses. The nurses prepared at the master's level also reported integrating more of the elements of the role as defined by the Canadian Nurses Association. These elements include clinician, consultant, educator, researcher, and leader.[23]

Additional key roles that CNSs play in today's health care include creating and sustaining excellence in clinical practice and supporting the attainment of magnet designation[3] and clear support for the instruction and full implementation of evidence-based practice.[24] Quality and safety initiatives are heavily influenced by CNSs in all aspects of care but it is the environment of process and systems level improvements where they can and do have the greatest impact.

It seems that despite the work done by CNS leaders, there is much work still to be done. The continued confusion in the enactment of the role by the CNSs themselves lends itself to a discrediting of the role by others or, worse, a usurping of the competencies by other declared roles.[25–27] Where there is a lack of clarity, it presents an opportunity to others to step in and take on elements of the role or the role in whole, thereby continuing the confusion.

THE FUTURE

Although the future looks bright, there are many areas of concern as we move toward the vision of the future presented by NACNS in 2007.[28] Through the implementation of the consensus model, the enactment of the ACA,[1] and full implementation of the suggestions within the IOM report,[2] as well as the movement of many institutions toward the doctor of nursing practice (DNP), CNSs will have many opportunities. The difficulty will be how the professional role moves through, around, and with the various changes that will need to come as time moves forward and not become fragmented or lose cohesion. It is a critical time in the continued development of the CNS.

Consensus Model

Historically, many CNS education programs were established to focus on the role of CNS and the specialty. CNSs would graduate from a master's program as a CNS in diabetes, emergency services, or perioperative specialties, to name just a few. The difficulty with this now is the new focus on population rather than specialty. Under the consensus model proposal, these programs will not meet the newly defined requirements for education within 1 of the 6 population foci.

To further complicate the issue in the past, certification was seen as a mark of excellence in CNS practice and not an expectation for entry to practice.[28] The consensus model requires certification as an entry to practice assessment.[4] In the early model of education, CNSs graduating from programs did not sit for certification examinations for 2 reasons: (1) they needed to have at least 3 years of clinical practice before they were eligible to sit for certification examinations in their area or (2) there was no examination for their specialty because of the limited numbers of graduates each year. Tests were not developed because they would not be considered psychometrically sound and legally defensible with the low numbers of graduates in the programs each year. As a result of the historic process for education of CNSs, there are schools with programs focused on role and specialty that currently do not meet the requirements of the consensus model. These schools will need to change the focus and adjust the educational requirements to fully meet the expectations of the consensus model. Changing a curriculum is no small feat and in some cases takes years. Full implementation of the consensus model is expected by 2015.[4]

There are also some specialties that do not fit into the existing certification examinations. The specialties previously identified would fit into the family across-the-lifespan population, however there are currently few, if any, educational programs preparing an across-the-lifespan CNS and no existing certification examination for the CNS population of individual/family across the lifespan.

The next step in correcting this problem is that at least 2 certification examinations will need to be developed to fill the current voids in population foci in the consensus model for the CNS role: individual/family across the life span and gender specific. This situation has created a looping discussion in that no examination will be developed until schools have graduated enough students to sit for the examinations that will allow the examination to be psychometrically sound and legally defensible and many schools have expressed concern about changing their curriculum until a certification test is developed for their students on graduation. Although this is a conundrum, good minds within the NACNS and from many other professional organizations are working on the problem. The stakes are too high to not resolve this issue. Many specialty populations of patients depend on CNSs to provide care that is specific to their needs, and it would be unacceptable to let these patients go without the expert level of care they need and deserve.

The next area of concern is the process of moving forward with the implementation of the regulatory changes proposed in the consensus model on a state-by-state basis. The consensus model clearly states that there needs to be a grandfathering of currently practicing APRNs that do not meet the educational or certification requirements of the new model. The issue is that not all states recognized CNSs in the past. If they were not recognized in the past, then they did not exist. The question many states are asking is how do you grandfather a group that was not previously recognized? If we look at the IOM report,[2] it clearly states that all nurses need to work to the full extent of their training and education. With that in mind, state boards of nursing need to move forward to ensure that all CNSs are recognized within the state and licensed as APRNs. The NACNS is taking the lead to assist CNSs as they work with their state boards of nursing and has developed a tool kit to help with the state-by-state implementations of the consensus model. The National Council of State Boards of Nursing has also developed tools for state boards of nursing. Both of these organizations are working together to ensure that all patients continue to have access to the specialty care they need and deserve.

The consensus model, even with its challenges, when fully and correctly implemented, can bring on one of the greatest advancements in CNS practice across the country. CNS programs must be able to prepare CNSs with the role and population while simultaneously maintaining specialty. Certification examinations must be developed for all population foci for CNSs so that the model can move forward and benefit all CNS specialties and the patients they serve. Once all states address the issue of grandfathering existing CNSs and license CNSs in a uniform manner, CNSs will be able to move from state to state and bring with them the rich practice environments and successes achieved in other states. Uniform licensure, accreditation, certification, and education of CNSs will be an improvement from the current approach. All APRNs will benefit from the consensus model because it adds to the legitimacy of all the roles. The consensus model firmly places all APRNs in a leading role for the future of health care.

The Affordable Care Act

Health care reform will require change based on the evidence. Change will be required to improve outcome while at the same time reducing overall cost to the health care system. CNSs are trained and educated to perform the specific kinds of system changes that are based on evidence and measured by outcomes. All 3 spheres of influence where CNSs work will require change (direct patient care, nursing practice, and systems).[5] CNSs are known to be change agents who base the changes made on evidence to improve the outcomes and to reduce cost.[29] There is no other health care professional more suited to lead health care reform than the CNS. Every institution that delivers health care would clearly benefit from the skills, insight, and knowledge that CNSs can bring during this tumultuous time in health care. If organizations are looking to come out of this process as a reformed, cost-effective deliverer of quality health care, CNSs are a vital member of the team that will get them the desired outcomes.

The IOM Report on the Future of Nursing

The IOM report contains recommendations that, if fully implemented, will transform nursing. The recommendation for nurses to work to the full extent of their training and education provides CNSs with an impetus to move forward in many areas that have been littered with roadblocks. The differences in how a CNS practices from state to state, city to city, and even institution to institution have been part of the problem. Practice changes that have improved patient outcomes do not transfer easily when those that are implementing the change have different practice opportunities and restrictions. Once all CNSs have the same authority to practice to the full extent of their training and education, systemic improvements in both direct care provided by CNSs and nursing care in its entirety can be accomplished through the actions and activities of CNSs.

The Doctor of Nursing Practice

Although the singular education path to the CNS role has long been the master's degree, additional options for doctoral education are now available, including the DNP. The DNP was introduced in 2004 by the American Association of Colleges of Nursing based on 13 recommendations with rationale supporting clinically focused doctoral-level preparation for APRNs.[30] The subsequent reaction to this doctoral degree from the academic and practice communities has been complex and somewhat controversial, in particular for the CNS.[31]

A primary area of controversy was the suggestion that state regulatory bodies mandate the DNP degree for all APRNs, with the suggested implementation date of 2015. To date, no state board has recommended or required the DNP degree, and neither educational program accreditation body, the Collegiate Center for Nursing Education or the National League for Nursing Accreditation Commission (NLN-AC), have stipulated that a DNP degree will be required for APRN graduates.[32,33] In addition, no professional certification body includes a DNP degree for certification eligibility. At present, no date has been established by the accrediting agencies for implementation of DNP requirements. In the authors' opinion, there will likely not be any date established for a mandated completion of the DNP. There are, however, 153 schools offering the DNP degree.[34]

Where CNSs are choosing to enroll in DNP programs, it is imperative that the program offers a CNS track. CNS is a distinct functional role, as are the other APRN roles (nurse practitioner, nurse midwife, and nurse anesthetist), and role competencies should be included in the graduate program. DNP programs that prepare CNSs for entry into advanced practice, (ie, bachelor of science in nursing [BSN]-DNP) must include CNS role competencies in the program and graduates must be eligible to sit for CNS certification examinations. Post–master of science in nursing (MSN) DNP programs that admit CNSs should offer doctoral-level CNS courses addressing the doctoral-level CNS competencies identified by the NACNS.[35]

Master's degree preparation remains an option for CNSs. Many schools of nursing have elected to maintain their master's degrees for entry into CNS practice. The National League for Nursing (NLN) issued a thoughtful white paper on the role of masters education[36] that affirms the value and credibility of both the MSN and DNP programs in today's health care system and supporting an inclusive model that does not devalue one program over another. The decision to offer MSN, BSN-DNP, or post-MSN DNP is one that schools need to carefully consider based on the needs of their home communities, faculty resources, and university/school configuration.[36] Some schools are unable to offer a doctoral degree because of the current level of approval for degree granting by the board of trustees/directors or perhaps even the charter of the school itself. The issues of the nursing faculty shortage and current overall economic climate are also important considerations for schools and potential students alike.

Also emerging is the BSN–doctor of philosophy option for CNSs. These programs will prepare graduates with a CNS role practice competencies and doctorate-level skills for knowledge generation. As nursing education continues to evolve, there may be other options. Most important to the advancement of the CNS role is the ability of any graduate program to embed the CNS practice competencies into the educational program. Where certification options are available, CNS programs should prepare students to meet certification eligibility requirements.

The 2015 date as a requirement for all CNSs to graduate with a DNP as entry into practice seems at best premature. In 2009, the NACNS took a neutral stance on the DNP,[37] indicating that the overall concept of advancing the educational level for CNSs was good but that there were many concerns as to the implementation. Since that time, the NACNS has published doctoral competences for CNS practice[35] and just released the educational criteria for both master's and doctoral education.[38] The NACNS continues to strongly support master's-level preparation as sufficient for entry to practice as a CNS as well as the value-added addition of doctoral-level preparation.

As CNS education moves forward, there are at the least 3 issues that need to remain front and center. These issues were raised in the 2005 NACNS white paper and again in the NLN document in 2010.[31,36] The first is the need for consensus as this or any other major initiative moves forward. The divisiveness and the energy wasted in public debate have reduced the ability for the nursing community to focus on the other issues that are impacting the nursing community as a whole. The second issue is a call for the data that demonstrate the need for a change. We are in a world that demands that data be generated to support any change being implemented, yet there seems to be a lack of evidence showing a difference in the outcomes of the MSN and the DNP APRN. Last but not least is the need to ensure that CNS doctoral competencies and education criteria are the foundation of any CNS DPN program.

None of the issues mentioned previously are insurmountable, and with a little thoughtful work, CNSs will be able to meet the requirements of the consensus model, the recommendations of the IOM report, the implementation of the DNP degree, and work to the fullest extent of their training and education and assist other personnel to do the same. The opportunities of the consensus model, the IOM report, health care reform, and the DNP degree far outweigh any challenges that have arisen to date.

SUMMARY

The CNS has a long and illustrious history. One can see its beginnings within the work of Florence Nightingale during the Crimean war.[6] In 1900, DeWitt[13] first described the concept of specialization, and in 1943, Reiter was talking about the expert "nurse-clinician".[7] In 1956, the NLN sponsored a conference on the education of the clinical specialist in psychiatric nursing and published the results of the conference in 1958.[14] The role was firmly established, competencies were developed for psychiatric CNSs, and other specialties were rapidly following. In 1995, a national organization for all CNS regardless of specialty was formed and began working on core competencies by 1996, with a first publication in 1998.[16] The final piece to cement the CNS role in society was the publication of the consensus model in 2008. This model outlined the requirements for licensure of CNSs, accreditation of education programs, certification of graduates, and education criteria. Through the subsequent work to implement the consensus model, CNSs will be able to address many of the issues, such as lack of uniformity and role confusion, that have previously plagued the role.

As stated earlier, the perfect storm is here: health care reform, the IOM report, and the consensus model have all come together at one time. These 3 opportunities, along with the proliferation of institutions seeking magnet status, place the demand for the CNS role at an all-time high. The stage is set, and all the players are in place. The opportunities for CNSs to lead the changes required to have legitimate reform are endless. The CNS is trained to lead change in 3 of the most impactful areas of health care: direct patient care, nursing practice, and systems. Over the next several years, the demand for the work of CNS will grow exponentially, which will place a strain on the already-burdened nursing education system. All 3.2 million nurses in the United States must arise and meet the challenges. By working together and drawing from within, we will be able to meet the needs of our patients now and into the future. This task is just one more job for the CNS. The future is bright, and the next act in this play seems to be starring the CNS.

REFERENCES

1. Patient Protection and Affordable Care Act – Public Law 111-148 (May 2011). Available at: http://docs.house.gov/energycommerce/ppacacon.pdf. Accessed October 22, 2011.

2. Institute of Medicine. The future of nursing. Author: National Academies Press; 2010. Available at: http://www.iom.edu/Reports/2010/The-Future-of-Nursing-Leading-Change-Advancing-Health.aspx. Accessed October 22, 2011.
3. Muller AC, Hujcs M, Dubendorf P, et al. Sustaining excellence: clinical nurse specialist practice and magnet designation. Clin Nurse Spec 2010;24(5):252–9.
4. APRN Joint Dialogue Group. Consensus model for APRN regulation: licensure, accreditation, certification & education: 2008. Available at: http://www.nacns.org/docs/APRN-RegulatoryModel.pdf. Accessed October 23, 2011.
5. Statement on practice and education of clinical nurse specialists. 2nd edition. Harrisburg (PA): National Association of Clinical Nurse Specialists; 2004.
6. Chinn P, Kramer M. Nursing knowledge development pathways. In: Theory and nursing: integrated knowledge development. 5th edition. St Louis (MO): Mosby; 1999. p. 17–47.
7. Reiter F. The nurse-clinician. Am J Nurs 1966;66:274–80.
8. Little D. The nurse specialist. Am J Nurs 1967;67:552–6.
9. Fulton J. Evolution of clinical nurse specialist role and practice in the United States. In: Fulton J, Lyon B, Goudreau K, editors. Foundations of clinical nurse specialist practice. New York: Springer; 2010. p. 3–13.
10. Sills G. The role and function of the clinical nurse specialist. In: Chaska NL, editor. The nursing profession: a time to speak. New York: McGraw-Hill; 1983. p. 563–79.
11. Statement on practice and education of clinical nurse specialists. Harrisburg (PA): National Association of Clinical Nurse Specialists; 1998.
12. Hiestand W. Frances U. Reiter and the graduate school of nursing at the New York College, 1960-1973. Nurs Hist Rev 2006;14:213–26.
13. DeWitt K. Specialties in nursing. Am J Nurs 2000;100(10):96AAA–96CCC.
14. Report of a national working conference: the education of the clinical specialist in psychiatric nursing. New York: National League for Nursing; 1958.
15. Social policy statement. Kanas City (MO): American Nurses Association; 1980.
16. Baldwin K, Lyon B, Clark A, et al. Developing clinical nurse specialist practice competencies. Clin Nurse Spec 2007;21(6):297–302.
17. A vision of the future of advanced practice registered nurse practice. Chicago: National Council of State Boards of Nursing; 2006.
18. National Clinical Nurse Specialist Competency Task Force. Clinical nurse specialist core competencies: executive summary 2006-2008. Harrisburg (PA): National Association of Clinical Nurse Specialists; 2010.
19. Fulton JS, Lyon BL, Goudreau KA. Foundations of clinical nurse specialist practice. New York: Springer Publishing Company; 2010.
20. Logical job analysis for clinical nurse specialist core examination. Summary report. Washington, DC: American Nurses Credentialing Center; 2008.
21. Lewandowski W, Adamle K. Substantive areas of clinical nurse specialist practice: a comprehensive review of the literature. Clin Nurse Spec 2009;23(2):73–90.
22. Bryant-Lukosious D. The clinical nurse specialist role in Canada: forecasting the future through research. Can J Nurs Res 2010;42(2):19–25.
23. Canadian Nurses Association (2009). Position statement: clinical nurse specialist. Available at: http://www.cna-aiic.ca/cna/documents/pdf/publications/ps104 clinical_nurse_specialist_e.pdf on. Accessed October 22, 2011.
24. Kring D. Clinical nurse specialist practice domains and evidence-based practice competencies: a matrix of influence. Clin Nurse Spec 2008;22(4):179–83.
25. Carol R. Something old, something new. Minority nurse, Summer 2009. Available at: http://www.minoritynurse.com/minority-nurse-leaders/something-old-something-new. Accessed October 22, 2011.

26. Goudreau K. Confusion, concern, or complimentary function: the overlapping roles of the clinical nurse specialist and the clinical nurse leader. Nurs Adm Q 2008;32(4):301–7.
27. Scott E, Cleary B. Professional polarities in nursing. Nurs Outlook 2007;55(5): 250–6.
28. Goudreau K, Baldwin K, Clark A, et al. A vision of the future for clinical nurse specialists. Harrisburg (PA): National Association of Clinical Nurse Specialists; 2007.
29. Newhouse R, Stanik-Hutt J, White K, et al. Advanced practice nurse outcomes 1990-2008: a systematic review. Nurs Econ 2011;29(5):1–22.
30. American Association of Colleges of Nursing. Position statement on the practice doctorate in nursing. Washington, DC: Author; 2004. Available at: http://www. aacn.nche.edu/DNP/DNPPositionStatement.htm. Accessed October 22, 2011.
31. NACNS. White paper on the nursing practice doctorate. 2005. Available at: http:// www.nacns.org/. Accessed October 22, 2011.
32. NLN-AC. NLN-AC statement on clinical practice doctorates. Available at: http:// www.nlnac.org/statementClinPrac.htm. Accessed October 22, 2011.
33. CCNE (2010) CCNE reaffirms commitment to accrediting all types of master' degree nursing programs. Available at: http://www.aacn.nche.edu/ccne-accreditation/ MSNletter.pdf. Accessed October 22, 2011.
34. 2010–2011 enrollment and graduations in baccalaureate and graduate programs in nursing. Washington, DC: American Nurses Credentialing Center; 2011.
35. National Association of Clinical Nurse Specialist. (2009) Core practice doctorate clinical nurse specialist (CNS) competencies. Available at: http://www.nacns.org/ docs/CorePracticeDoctorate.pdf. Accessed October 22, 2011.
36. National League for Nursing. (2010) Master's education in nursing. Available at: http://www.nln.org/aboutnln/reflection_dialogue/refl_dial_6.htm. Accessed October 22, 2011.
37. National Association of Clinical Nurse Specialist. (2009) Position statement on the practice nursing doctorate. Available at: http://www.nacns.org/docs/ PositionOnNursingPracticeDoctorate.pdf. Accessed October 22, 2011.
38. National Association of Clinical Nurse Specialist. (2012) Criteria for the evaluation of clinical nurse specialist master's, practice doctorate, and post-graduate certificate educational programs. Available at: http://www.nacns.org. Accessed October 22, 2011.

Nurse-Midwifery: Art and Science

Debora M. Dole, PhD, CNM, RN*,
Cynthia F. Nypaver, MSN, CNM, WHNP-BC

KEYWORDS

- Nurse midwifery • Women's health • Health disparities
- Advanced practice registered nurse

KEY POINTS

- Midwives share a rich history with nursing and midwifery, and a shared commitment to the health of people across the lifespan.
- In a difficult economic, social, and political landscape, health disparities continue to widen.
- Advanced practice registered nurses (APRNs), including nurse-midwives, have demonstrated an ability to rise to the occasion when challenged, and caring for the disadvantaged in a difficult health care environment is such an occasion.

The gap in the health of the nations' people seems to be widening and reflects existing social inequalities affecting the ongoing health of individuals. Healthy People 2010 has come and gone—its goals mostly unmet. More people of color continue to die from a wide range of health conditions across all age ranges and income levels compared to whites.[1] Healthy People 2020 is on the horizon with a wide range of objectives from access to health services to identifying the impact of social determinants of health.[2] The objectives are designed to address and eliminate health disparities as well as improve the health of all individuals. Recent health care reform focuses on improving quality and reducing cost by promoting interdisciplinary and interprofessional health care teams.[3,4] Nursing, particularly advanced practice nursing, is positioned to meet the challenge and make a difference. From a historical and practical perspective, certified nurse-midwives (CNMs) are one group of APRNs uniquely situated to address existing disparities related to maternal-child health. This article provides an overview of the historical development, current status, and use of CNMs in the United States health care system; the impact of CNMs on maternal-child health outcomes; and future trends in the education of CNMs.

University of Cincinnati, College of Nursing, Academic Health Center, PO Box 210038, Cincinnati, OH 45221-0038, USA
* 1225 Carolina Trace Road, West Harrison, IN 47060.
E-mail address: Debora.dole@gmail.com

Nurs Clin N Am 47 (2012) 205–213
doi:10.1016/j.cnur.2012.02.008
0029-6465/12/$ – see front matter © 2012 Elsevier Inc. All rights reserved.

NURSE-MIDWIFERY: A HYPHENATED HISTORY

Historically speaking, nursing and midwifery have not always coexisted as a single discipline. Nursing and midwifery are two distinct bodies of knowledge that bring together the art and science of caring for women across the lifespan. The term nurse-midwife is uniquely American. In most areas of the world, midwifery practice is viewed as an independent profession separate from nursing and governed by a variety of central governing boards that include boards of midwifery (Ireland and the United Kingdom) and dual governing boards of nursing and midwifery (Australia).[5] Midwifery practice as defined by the American College of Nurse Midwives (ACNM) is the independent management of women's health care including primary care, family planning, pregnancy, childbearing, and menopause by certified midwives (CMs) and CNMs.[6,7] It is important to understand the distinction. Both CNMs and CMs must pass the same national certification examination administered by the American Midwifery Certification Board, the independent national certifying body for midwifery practice. CNMs are educated in the two disciplines of nursing and midwifery at the master's level (eg, Master of Science, Master Public Health) or doctoral level (eg, Doctor of Public Health, Doctor of Philosophy, Doctor of Nursing Practice). CMs are educated at the master's or doctoral level in the discipline of midwifery.[6,7]

Conflict over the professional identity of nurse-midwives is evident in that some within the profession self-identify as midwives with a nursing background and others self-identify as nurses with advanced training in midwifery. To understand the split identity, it is important to also understand the historical significance of the union. In 1911, a resolution proposed by Lillian Wald to educate American nurses in midwifery failed at the American Association for the Study and Prevention of Infant Mortality. In 1955, the National League for Nursing (NLN) and the American Nurses Association (ANA) refused to recognize nurse-midwifery practice as nursing practice.[8–11] Nurse-midwives have continued to identify themselves as autonomous practitioners with a distinct and shared history. **Table 1** provides a timeline for the parallel evolution of nurse-midwifery practice and nurse-midwifery education. The evolution of nurse-midwifery practice has always been reflected in nurse-midwifery education, which has been quick to respond to current and anticipated needs of an ever-changing health landscape.[11]

Mary Breckenridge is credited with bringing midwifery to nursing in the form of a hybrid practitioner educated in nursing and midwifery. Breckenridge started the Frontier Nursing Service in rural Kentucky in 1925, the first nurse-midwifery clinical service in the United States.[9] Frontier Nursing Service, as the sole provider of health care for families living in rural Kentucky, was credited with dramatically improving the dismal infant mortality rate as well as improving health for entire families.[9,10] Breckenridge was also credited with creating the Kentucky State Association of Midwives, which eventually become the American Association of Nurse-Midwives. Its purpose was to develop recommendations and standards for midwifery practice, certification, and education.[9–11] The ACNM was founded in 1955 as a result of the rejection, by the NLN and the ANA, of the request for an autonomous council to represent the concerns of nurse-midwives within either organization.[9] With the creation of the ACNM, the professional identity of nurse-midwives was solidified as separate and apart from nursing—a unique hybrid.[8,12]

Since 1955, the ACNM has evolved into a professional organization responsible for setting practice standards, developing core competencies for basic midwifery education, accreditation of educational programs, monitoring certification of midwives (CMs) and nurse-midwives (CNMs), professional development, political action, and policy development. The ACNM also publishes a variety of professional publications, including the *Journal of Midwifery and Women's Health* and other resources directed at the business of midwifery, and it provides public outreach and education.[7,13,14]

NURSE-MIDWIFERY CARE: USE AND IMPACT ON PATIENT OUTCOMES

Fifty percent of all babies born in the United States were born into the hands of a midwife at the turn of the twentieth century.[8,10] By 1930, the number of midwife-attended births had decreased to 15% primarily due to the medicalization of birth by obstetricians seeking to develop the medical specialty and eliminate traditional midwives. The midwives, who served primarily poor immigrant populations, were unfairly categorized as uneducated and dangerous.[10] Even though the campaign to eliminate the traditional midwife was largely successful, the value of midwifery care was not lost on those public health officials and activists who sought to have nurses trained in midwifery. The impact of nurse-midwives on maternal and infant health outcomes has long been recognized. Breckinridge documented the direct effect of nurse-midwifery care on the maternal mortality rate in Appalachia by enlisting the Metropolitan Life Insurance Company to assist her in collecting data on over 10,000 births over a 30-year period.[9,10] The maternal mortality rate for midwife-attended births in 1927 was less than half the rate of physician-attended births (51 maternal deaths per 10,000 live births vs 111 deaths per 10,000 live births, respectively).[9,10]

Continued competition, third-party insurance payers, and the continually changing social context of birth and women's health care have had an effect on the growth of midwifery over the past several decades. In 2009, CNMs attended 11.3% of the vaginal births and 7.6% of total births in the United States.[15,16] The goal of the American College of Nurse-Midwives is that CNMs and CMs will attend 20% of all births in the United States by 2020.[16] Midwifery care has been viewed as particularly useful in underserved communities where populations were vulnerable to poor health due to low income, minority race, immigrant status, or access to care limited by either available physician providers or distance to facilities.[17,18] Historically, restrictive state laws existed insuring midwives could only practice in areas where physicians were in short supply.[17] In part due to improved outcomes directly related to midwifery care and consumer demands for personalized and high quality care, that view is changing. Midwifery services are expanding into private practice settings, community-based health centers, academic health centers, and private hospitals.

Midwifery care has long been associated with cost-effective care. The midwifery philosophy of care incorporates a belief in equal access to care. The philosophy incorporates a partnership approach that supports self-determination, active participation, and nonintervention in normal process with appropriate use of interventions and technology when necessary.[6,15] Although midwives provide the same standard of care expected by all providers, the judicious use of technology and intervention when indicated has been shown to lower the overall cost of care delivered without compromising quality or outcomes.[18–21] Optimal perinatal care has been defined by Kennedy[19] as "the maximal perinatal outcome with minimal intervention placed against the context of the women's social, medical, and obstetric history." In an era in which cost-benefit is of concern to everyone, the ability of CNMs to provide high quality, cost-effective care has been recognized as beneficial to women as well as institutions.

Midwifery's commitment to providing woman-focused care can be seen in the development and implementation of group prenatal care. Centering Pregnancy is an innovative approach to providing prenatal care that is changing the way prenatal

Table 1
Timeline of critical events in nurse-midwifery practice and nurse-midwifery education

Date	Midwifery Profession	Midwifery Education
1911	Lillian Wald introduced resolution to educate American nurses in midwifery at the American Association for the Study and Prevention of Infant Mortality; resolution not adopted	—
1914	Introduced title "nurse-midwife" to differentiate from traditional immigrant midwives	Dr Fred Taussig called for the education of nurses in midwifery at the annual meeting of NOPHN
1918	Maternity Center Association established in New York City to promote family-centered maternity care with a public health focus	—
1922	—	Dr Ralph Lobestine suggested in the *American Journal of Public Health* that educating nurses to manage normal labor would reduce infant mortality
1924	Public health nurse, Mary Beard, RN, sent by the Rockefeller Foundation to study the "relations of midwifery to nursing."	—
1925	Mary Breckenridge opened FNS, the first nurse-midwifery clinical service in the United States	Manhattan Midwifery School opened first program to educate registered nurses in midwifery
1929	Kentucky State Association of Midwives founded by Mary Breckenridge	—
1931	Lobestine Midwifery Clinic in New York City was the second midwifery service to open (Hattie Hemschemeyer, director)	—
1932	—	Lobestine Midwifery School opened second education program for nurse-midwives
1939	—	FNS opened third education program for nurse-midwives
1940	Hemschemeyer convened the National Association of Certified Nurse-Midwives to represent and provide guidance for education programs and practice	—

1940	Kentucky State Association of Midwives became the American Association of Nurse-Midwives	—
1942	First nurse-midwifery operated "birthing center" opened in rural Georgia supported by the Georgia Department of Health	—
1944	Hemschemeyer formed an autonomous nurse-midwifery section within NOPHN; first nurse-midwifery organization open to nurses of color (disbanded in 1952 with the dissolution of the NOPHN)	—
1947	—	Catholic University of America granted the first Master of Science degree with a Certificate in Nurse-Midwifery
1953	First nurse-midwifery service in an academic medical center opened at Johns Hopkins	Nurse-midwifery education program at Johns Hopkins funded
1955	ACNM founded as a result of NLN and ANA refusal to acknowledge nurse-midwifery as nursing practice	—
1962	ACNM approved definition of the nurse-midwife and nurse-midwifery practice	Criteria for Evaluation of Nurse-Midwifery Programs approved
1966	ACNM approved and published "Function, Standards, and Qualifications for the Practice of Nurse-Midwifery"	—
1969	American Association of Nurse-Midwives merged with ACNM	—
1971	National certification examination established by ACNM	—
1978	—	Core Competencies for Nurse-Midwifery Education issued (revised, 1985, 1992, 1997, 2002, 2010)
1989	—	FNS School became the Community-Based Nurse-Midwifery Education Program, the first distance-learning midwifery education program
1996	—	ACNM Division of Accreditation approved education standards for preparation and certification for the CM

Abbreviations: FNS, Frontier Nursing Service; NOPHN, National Organization for Public Health Nurses.
Adapted from Refs.[9-11]

care is being delivered nation-wide. Centering Pregnancy is a group model of prenatal care developed to incorporate assessment, education, social support, and self-empowerment.[22,23] Implementation of the Centering Pregnancy model of care has demonstrated improved health outcomes for childbearing women and their infants that includes significant decreases in low birth-weight babies, preterm birth, as well as significant increases in breastfeeding rates, prenatal knowledge, and readiness for labor and delivery.[22–26] In addition, women demonstrate high satisfaction with group prenatal care.[27] The old saying "When mama is happy, everyone is happy" seems to ring true to for this model of care, including mom, fetus, practitioner, and policymakers.

Innovation and a commitment to providing culturally sensitive care to the most vulnerable that is evidenced-based are hallmarks of midwifery care. Generations of women and their families have benefited from this ongoing commitment. Continued efforts to collaborate, communicate, and educate will undoubtedly provide future generations with improved access to health care uniquely suited to meet their needs.

WHAT DOES THE FUTURE LOOK LIKE?

The future demands a health care system that is responsive to the needs of a population in a constantly changing environment. Nurse-midwives share a history that combines the strengths, art, and science of nursing with the tradition of midwifery. APRNs can begin by shifting the focus from a biomedical model of care to a more holistic model of care that is consistent with nursing and midwifery philosophy. Recent federal legislation has identified access, quality, and cost as primary objectives necessary for improvement of the health care system.[3] Nurse-midwives have already demonstrated an ability to improve access, deliver high quality care, and reduce cost. It would seem that we are prepared to meet the challenge.

PROFESSIONAL TRENDS

The ACNM, the Accreditation Commission for Midwifery Education, and the American Midwifery Certification Board are committed to promoting the "Consensus Model for APRN Regulation" as it applies to midwifery practice with special considerations for the scope of midwifery practice.[28] Standardization of APRN licensures, accreditation, certification, and education based on the principle of APRN practice autonomy is consistent with midwifery standards already in place.[29]

The ACNM defines midwifery practice as the independent management of women's health care in which midwives collaborate and consult when indicated.[6] Practice autonomy is essential to the effective implementation of the Consensus Model for midwifery practice and APRNs.[28] Supervisory language and collaborative agreement requirements represent needless barriers to APRN practice and access to health care services while providing no benefits in quality of care.[28] Collegial relationships characterized by mutual respect, trust, professional responsibility, and accountability enhance quality of care but sometimes can be challenging.[29] Artificial limits placed on practice autonomy (eg, scope of practice, prescriptive authority, and practice location) only serve to further divide, inhibit access, and reduce quality of care.

EDUCATION

The discipline of midwifery has a long and rich history of caring for women and their families with an emphasis on improving health outcomes. To develop leadership knowledge, skills, and competencies that foster changes to improve health care for women and their families, the profession is called on to expand opportunities for education at the highest levels of midwifery practice. The ACNM currently endorses the master's degree as basic preparation for midwifery practice and recognizes the need to develop competencies for midwifery education at the doctoral level.[30] The ACNM also supports a variety of doctoral degree options for midwives.[30] The ACNM also is responsible for ensuring that the midwifery body of knowledge is clearly represented in the Doctor of Nursing Practice curriculum that includes a solid foundation of leadership knowledge, skills, and competencies necessary to assess and improve health care processes and outcomes.[30]

To meet the demand for health care providers, educational programs need to evaluate their ability to produce qualified, prepared professionals.[31] Along with levels of educational preparation are the various formats in which curricula are delivered. To meet the CNMs goal of 1000 newly certified CNMs by 2015, an average increase of 25% growth over the next 3 years will be needed.[16] The combination of numbers of midwifery education programs, student capacity, preceptor availability, midwifery faculty, and qualified applicants requires a complex roadmap to attain the goal of increasing the numbers of CNMs. Distance education has improved access for many future CNMs. Frontier School of Nursing's Community-Based Nursing Education Program pioneered the distance learning format for nurse-midwifery education in 1990 by providing students with concentrated learning modules combined with on-site intensive learning labs, followed by clinical application performed via clinical preceptors in the student's local community. Currently, a wide range of distance learning options is available for students.

The Midwifery Education Trends Report for 2011 cites the following recommendations for increasing the number of CNMs to meet the projected need[16]:

- Increase number of accelerated or second degree registered nurse plus APRN programs
- Develop new education programs for the preparation of CM in schools of nursing and/or allied health
- Support and train preceptors
- Support increased funding for basic and graduate nursing education.

Regardless of the educational path chosen, all graduates must graduate from an accredited program, attain basic competency as determined by the ACNM Core Competencies for Basic Midwifery Practice, and pass the national certifying examination. The process is designed to ensure a qualified and competent base from which to begin midwifery practice.

SUMMARY

We are poised to continue in the tradition of our foremothers. Midwives share a rich history with nursing and midwifery. Both disciplines have demonstrated a commitment to improving the health of people across the lifespan, especially those at the greatest risk for poor health outcomes. Even so, health disparities continue to exist. The gap continues to widen. The shifting political and social landscape often serves to complicate an already complex system that further disadvantages those who can afford to lose the least. APRNs, including nurse-midwives, have demonstrated an ability to rise to the occasion when challenged. Challenge and opportunity can seem quite similar at times. This one looks like both. Understanding the past has implications for preparing for the future. We are prepared.

REFERENCES

1. MacDorman MF, Mathews TJ. CDC Health Disparities and Inequalities Report—United States, 2011. MMWR Surveill Summ 2011. Available at: http://www.cdc.gov/mmwr/pdf/other/su6001.pdf. Accessed February 1, 2011.
2. Healthy People 2020 topics & objectives. US Department of Health and Human Services; 2011. Available at: http://healthypeople.gov/2020/topicsobjectives2020/default.aspx. Accessed December 10, 2011.
3. Martinez J, Ro M, Villa NW, et al. Transforming the delivery of care in the post-health reform era: what role will community health workers play? Am J Public Health 2011;101(12):e1–5.
4. Farley T. Reforming health care or reforming health? Am J Public Health 2009;4(9):588–90.
5. Australian Nursing and Midwifery Council. National competency standards for the midwife. Nursing and Midwifery Board of Australia; 2006. Available at: http://www.nursingmidwiferyboard.gov.au/Codes-Guidelines-Statements/Codes-Guidelines.aspx. Accessed December 10, 2011.
6. American College of Nurse-Midwives. Definition of midwifery practice. Position statement. ACNM Standard Setting Documents. 2004. Available at: http://www.midwife.org/siteFiles/position/Def_of_Mid_Prac_CNM_CM_05.pdf. Accessed October 4, 2011.
7. American College of Nurse-Midwives. Core competencies for basic midwifery practice. 2008. Available at: http://www.midwife.org. Accessed December 10, 2011.
8. Dawley K. American nurse-midwifery: A hyphenated profession with a conflicted identity. Nsg History Review 2005;13:147–70.
9. Dawley K, Varney Burst H. The American College of Nurse-Midwives and its antecedents: a historic time line. J Midwifery Womens Health 2005;50:16–22.
10. Dawley K. Origins of nurse-midwifery in the United States and its expansion in the 1940s. J Midwifery Womens Health 2003;48:86–95.
11. Varney Burst H. The history of nurse-midwifery/midwifery education. J Midwifery Womens Health 2005;50(2):129–37.
12. Varney Burst H. Nurse-midwifery self-identification and autonomy. J Midwifery Womens Health 2005;55(5):406–10.
13. Avery M. The history and evolution of the core competencies for basic midwifery practice. J Midwifery Womens Health 2005;50(2):102–7.
14. Accreditation Commission for Midwifery Education (ACME). The knowledge, skills, and behaviors prerequisite to midwifery clinical coursework. Silver Spring (MD): Accreditation Commission for Midwifery Education (ACME); 2005.
15. American College of Nurse-Midwives. ACNM Position Statement. May 2011. Available at: http://www.Midwife.org. Accessed December 10, 2011.
16. Midwifery Education Trends Report 2011. ACNM. Silver Springs: ACNM, 2011. Available at: http://www.midwife.org/ACNM/files/ccLibraryFiles/FILENAME/000000001457/acnm%20midwiferyedtrend2011%20report%20011112.pdf. Accessed January 11, 2012.
17. Raisler J, Kennedy H. Midwifery care of poor and vulnerable women, 1925-2003. J Midwifery Womens Health 2005;50(2):113–21.
18. Kennedy HP, Shannon MT, Chuahorm U, et al. The landscape of caring for women: a narrative study of midwifery practice. J Midwifery Womens Health 2004;49(1):14–23.
19. Kennedy HP. A concept analysis of "optimality" in perinatal health. JOGNN 2006;35:763–9.

20. Cragin L, Kennedy HP. Linking obstetric and midwifery practice with optimal outcomes. JOGNN 2006;35(6):779–85.

21. Doherty ME. Midwifery care: reflections of midwifery clients. J Perinatal Education 2010;19(4):41–51.

22. Alexander G, Kotelchuck M. Assessing the role and effectiveness of prenatal care: history, challenges, and directions for future research. Public Health Rep 2001;306–16.

23. Carlson N, Lowe N. Centering pregnancy: a new approach in prenatal care. MCN Am J Matern Child Nurs 2006;31(4):218–23.

24. Baldwin K. Comparison of selected outcomes of centering pregnancy versus traditional prenatal care. J Midwifery Womens Health 2006;51(4):266–72.

25. Ickovics J, Kershaw T, Westdahl C, et al. Group prenatal care and perinatal outcomes: a randomized controlled trial. Obstet Gynecol 2007;110(2 pt 1):330–9.

26. Novick G. Women's experience of prenatal care: an integrative review. J Midwifery Womens Health 2009;54(3):226–37.

27. Novick G, Sadler LS, Kennedy HP, et al. Women's experience of group prenatal care. Qualitative Health Research 2011;21(1):97–116.

28. American College of Nurse-Midwives (ACNM), Accreditation Commission for Midwifery Education (ACME), American Midwifery Certification Board (AMCB). Midwifery in the United States and the Consensus Model for APRN Regulation. 2011. Midwife.org/ACNM Library. Available at: http://www.midwife.org/index.asp?bid=59&cat=12&button=Search&rec=254. Accessed December 10, 2011.

29. Kennedy HP. Tensions and teamwork in nursing and midwifery relationships. JOGNN 2008;37:426–35.

30. American College of Nurse-Midwives. Midwifery education and the doctor of nursing practice (DNP) position statement. 2011. Available at: http://www.midwife.org/ACNM/files/ACNMLibraryData/IPLAODFILENAME/000000000079/Midwifery%20Ed%20and%20DNP%207.09.pdf. Accessed October 4, 2011.

31. Fagerlund K, Germano E. The costs and benefits of Nurse-Midwifery education: model and application. J Midwifery Womens Health 2009;54(5):341–50.

Nurse Anesthesia
A Past, Present, and Future Perspective

Wanda O. Wilson, CRNA, PhD, MSN

KEYWORDS

- Anesthesia • CRNAs • Health care reform • Advanced practice registered nurse

KEY POINTS

- The US health system is rapidly reaching a point at which inefficient use of resources and duplication of efforts cannot be sustained.
- The Institute of Medicine's 2010 report on the "Future of Nursing" clearly identified that the United States needs to examine how to make best use of highly qualified advanced practice registered nurses (APRNs) to drive a more efficient and effective health care system.
- Certified registered nurse anesthetists (CRNAs) will help manage this change by continuing to provide patient access to safe, cost-effective anesthesia care; knowing the direction in which health care is headed; being politically active at the state and federal levels; educating the public about the value of nurse anesthetists; and being involved at the local community and institutional levels.

The health care specialty of nurse anesthesia was born amid the battlefields of the American Civil War.

In 2012, some 150 years later, more than 44,000 CRNAs and student registered nurse anesthetists across the United States will administer approximately 32 million anesthetics to patients in every type of practice setting in which anesthesia is required. In addition, in testament to the profession's roots, today's nurse anesthetists remain the primary anesthesia caregivers to US service men and women at home and abroad.

Throughout their history, nurse anesthetists have prevailed over challenges from organized medicine and others who have sought to limit their scope of practice and reduce patient access to their services. Similar challenges lie ahead as the overburdened US health system turns to APNs and other specialists who are not medical doctors (MDs) or doctors of osteopathy (DOs), to fulfill a larger role in providing safe, cost-effective health care services to an aging patient population. Answering the call just as their forebears did during anesthesia's formative years, today's nurse anesthetists have embraced the responsibility of helping meet America's growing

Dedicated to John F. Garde, CRNA, MS, FAAN.
American Association of Nurse Anesthetists, 222 South Prospect Avenue, Park Ridge, IL 60068, USA
E-mail address: wwilson@aana.com

Nurs Clin N Am 47 (2012) 215–223
doi:10.1016/j.cnur.2012.02.010
0029-6465/12/$ – see front matter © 2012 Elsevier Inc. All rights reserved.

health care needs as well as the requirement of doctoral education for entry into nurse anesthesia practice by 2025, thereby ensuring patients continued access to the highest quality anesthesia care possible.

This article offers a brief history of nurse anesthesia, assesses the present state of the profession, and discusses why nurse anesthetists will continue to be an invaluable part of the US health care system well into the future.

A HISTORY OF MOVING FORWARD

With the discovery of the anesthetizing properties of various drugs during the mid–nineteenth century, the idea of using general anesthesia for surgery gained rapid popularity. However, having no one qualified to administer anesthetic agents, the job of anesthetist was passed to whoever was available, from house officers to medical students to janitors. As a result, anesthesia was cited as the cause of the greatest incidence of surgical morbidity and mortality in the late 1800s.

As the furor over the high death rate grew, surgeons decided that the major cause of the adverse effects of anesthesia was the so-called occasional anesthetist, and called for clinicians who would dedicate themselves solely to the specialty of anesthesia. In *History of Anesthesia with Emphasis on the Nurse Specialist* (1953), historian Virginia Thatcher identified the reasons why surgeons turned to nurses. According to Thatcher, surgeons "wanted a person who would (1) be satisfied with the subordinate role that the work required, (2) make anesthesia their one absorbing interest, (3) not look on the situation of anesthetist as one that put them in a position to watch and learn from the surgeon's technique, (4) accept relatively low pay, and (5) have the natural aptitude and intelligence to develop a high level of skill in providing the smooth anesthesia and relaxation that the surgeon demanded."

The earliest recorded nurse anesthetist was Sister Mary Bernard, a Catholic nun who administered anesthesia at St. Vincent's Hospital in Erie, Pennsylvania, in 1877. In the next 10 to 15 years, nurses made great progress as anesthesia providers with the support of pioneering physicians such as Dr William Worrall Mayo and his son, Dr Charles H. Mayo. Charles shared his father's belief that nurses were capable of becoming fine anesthetists, and in 1893 began working with Alice Magaw, who earned international respect and was given the title the Mother of Anesthesia by Charles for her outstanding performance and contributions to anesthesia. In December 1906, Magaw published "A Review of Over 14,000 Surgical Anesthetics" in *Surgery, Gynecology, and Obstetrics*. In the article, she reported using chloroform and ether anesthesia with the open-drop technique without a single fatality attributable to anesthesia.

The Mayo Clinic in Rochester, Minnesota, subsequently became a place where surgeons sent their nurses to observe and learn anesthesia administration from Magaw. Nurse anesthetists such as Magaw perfected the technique of using a combination of chloroform and ether by the open-drop method, which satisfied the surgeons and provided comfort and safety for their patients.

Another physician who greatly supported nurse anesthetists was Dr George Washington Crile at Lakeside Hospital in Cleveland, Ohio. In 1908, Crile asked Agatha Hodgins to become his personal anesthetist, and within a year she perfected the administration of nitrous oxide-oxygen anesthesia. Surgeons who came to observe both surgery and anesthesia at Lakeside were so impressed by this method of anesthesia that they asked to have nurses from their own clinics trained by Hodgins.

In 1915, on returning to the United States after providing care to wounded soldiers during World War I, Hodgins and Crile were faced with the first major challenge concerning nurses' rights to administer anesthesia. The Ohio State Medical Board sent a letter to Crile informing him that it was the board's decision that no one other than a registered physician was permitted to administer anesthesia, and that the state Attorney General concurred. The board also issued a cease-and-desist order to Crile, stating that, if he continued to use nurses in the administration of anesthesia, Lakeside Hospital's School of Nursing would lose its accreditation. It took 2 years for Crile to persuade the medical board to lift the order, and he and Hodgins began educating nurses in anesthesia once again. Crile and some of his supporters suspected that the same challenge could be directed at others; they went to the Ohio legislature to acquire an exemption within the Medical Practice Act for nurses appropriately educated in anesthesia to administer anesthesia under the supervision of a physician. This exemption was achieved in 1919, the first such mention of nurse anesthetists in a state statute.

Because of the many accomplishments of America's nurse anesthetists in front-line surgical units and hospitals during World War I, the demand for nurse anesthetists increased rapidly after the war. As a result, new nurse anesthesia educational programs moved into university hospitals and major community hospitals. During this period of growth for the profession, another serious challenge to nurse anesthesia practice arose when the Kentucky Medical Society alleged in 1917 that only physicians should administer anesthesia. With the concurrence of the state Attorney General, the society issued an ethical policy that sanctioned by expulsion any member of the society who used nurse anesthetists or practiced in hospitals that employed nurse anesthetists. Dr Louis Frank, a Louisville surgeon, and his nurse anesthetist, Margaret Hatfield, along with the Kentucky State Department of Health, filed suit against the society. Frank and Hatfield won at the appellate level, with the justice ruling that Hatfield was not practicing medicine in the way and under the circumstances in which she was administering anesthesia (Frank et al v. South et al, Kentucky Rep. 175:416–428).

The last significant court challenge on the subject of whether nurse anesthetists were practicing medicine came between 1933 and 1936, when Dagmar Nelson was charged by some physician anesthetists with such practice. Although the case went all the way to the California Supreme Court, favorable rulings for Nelson were rendered at each level (Chalmers-Francis et al v. Nelson et al (Calif) 57 P(2d) 1312).

Many important advances in practice rights and patient safety have been made by nurse anesthetists through the years, and although unnecessary challenges by the medical community have persisted, CRNAs and their professional organization, the American Association of Nurse Anesthetists (AANA), have been equally persistent in fending them off. In Bahn v NME Hospitals (1985), the US Circuit Court of Appeals ruled that, under certain circumstances, CRNAs working with physicians other than anesthesiologists can compete with anesthesiologists and thus have standing to bring a federal antitrust suit under circumstances prescribed in antitrust law. Nearly 2 decades later, in 2004, the Minnesota Association of Nurse Anesthetists (MANA) successfully resolved legal actions brought by MANA on behalf of the Federal Government against hospitals and anesthesiologists alleging wrongful termination of nurses, antitrust violations, and Medicare fraud. The lawsuit, which took 10 years to run its course, was instrumental in bringing about substantial regulatory changes regarding reimbursement of CRNAs and anesthesia professionals generally. Between these 2 important cases, Medicare direct reimbursement legislation for CRNAs was signed into law by President Ronald Reagan in 1986, making nurse anesthesia the first nursing specialty to be accorded direct reimbursement rights under this federal program.

NURSE ANESTHESIA IN THE TWENTY-FIRST CENTURY: SAFE, COST-EFFECTIVE ANESTHESIA CARE

The AANA today represents a profession that is more than 44,000 strong, including CRNAs and student registered nurse anesthetists. These APNs serve in various capacities in their daily practices, taking on roles of clinician, educator, administrator, manager, researcher, and consultant. The AANA establishes evidence-based professional standards of anesthesia care and guidelines for nurse anesthesia practice that are updated frequently, published in the *Professional Practice Manual*, and can be found online at www.aana.com.

CRNAs administer anesthesia for all types of surgical cases, use all anesthetic techniques, and practice in every setting in which anesthesia is delivered, including traditional hospital surgical suites and obstetric delivery rooms; critical access hospitals; ambulatory surgical centers; the offices of dentists, podiatrists, ophthalmologists, plastic surgeons, and pain management specialists; and US military, Public Health Services, and Department of Veterans Affairs health care facilities. They provide anesthesia in collaboration with surgeons, anesthesiologists, dentists, podiatrists, and other qualified health care professionals. When anesthesia is administered by a nurse anesthetist, it is recognized as the practice of nursing; when administered by an anesthesiologist, it is recognized as the practice of medicine. Regardless of whether their educational background is in nursing or medicine, all anesthesia professionals give anesthesia the same way. CRNAs provide services as employees of hospitals or physicians or as private practitioners either by clinical privileging and/or as contractors; the average annual compensation for a CRNA is approximately $160,000.

CRNAs are the sole anesthesia professionals in most rural hospitals in the United States, and, in some states, are the sole anesthesia professionals in nearly 100% of rural facilities. CRNAs also provide a significant percentage of anesthesia care in inner cities and other medically underserved areas of the United States, affording patients in these areas access to essential surgical, obstetric, trauma stabilization, and pain management services.

Landmark Studies Confirm CRNA Safety and Cost-Effectiveness

At the turn of this century, major regulatory events were taking place that would profoundly change the health care landscape for nurse anesthetists and their patients. In 1997, the Health Care Financing Administration (HCFA; now the Centers for Medicare & Medicaid Services [CMS]) of the Department of Health and Human Services released a proposed rule to defer to the states on physician supervision of CRNAs for Medicare cases. With the announcement, the AANA made this its top legislative and regulatory priority, as did the American Society of Anesthesiologists (ASA), which was determined to prevent the removal of this outdated reimbursement requirement. The issue was vigorously debated in Washington, DC, state capitals, and the media for 3 years before the HCFA announced in 2000 that it would finalize the rule removing the federal requirement and deferring to the states on physician supervision of CRNAs for Medicare cases. Because the rule was published in the *Federal Register* in the last days of the Clinton administration, it was delayed by the new Bush administration and reconsidered. Subsequently, a different rule was published in November 2001 that kept in place the Medicare requirement of physician supervision of CRNAs while establishing a process by which state governors could write to CMS to opt out of the requirement. Less than 1 month after finalization of the supervision opt-out rule, Iowa became the first state to take advantage of the opportunity to remove the physician supervision requirement for nurse anesthetists working in that state. Since then,

15 states have followed Iowa's lead, bringing to 16 the number of states that no longer require physician supervision of nurse anesthetists.

When the final rule was published, CMS expressed interest in an eventual study on anesthesia safety in the states where physician supervision was no longer required. Nine years later, in 2010, researchers from RTI International examined nearly 500,000 individual Medicare cases in the first 14 opt-out states and concluded that "there are no differences in patient outcomes when anesthesia services are provided by Certified Registered Nurse Anesthetists (CRNAs), physician anesthesiologists, or CRNAs supervised by physicians." This landmark study, titled "No Harm Found When Nurse Anesthetists Work Without Supervision by Physicians," was published in the August issue of *Health Affairs*. Also in 2010, another important study, this one conducted by The Lewin Group and published in the *Journal of Nursing Economic$*, determined that a CRNA "acting as the sole anesthesia provider is the most cost effective model of anesthesia delivery." This study, titled "Cost Effectiveness Analysis of Anesthesia Providers," considered the different anesthesia delivery models in use in the United States today, including CRNAs acting solo, physician anesthesiologists acting solo, and various models in which a single anesthesiologist directs or supervises 1 to 6 CRNAs. The results showed that CRNAs acting as the sole anesthesia provider cost 25% less than the second lowest cost model. The Lewin researchers also conducted a thorough review of the literature that compares the quality of anesthesia service by provider type or delivery model, and determined that the published studies show that there are no measurable differences in the quality of care between CRNAs and anesthesiologists or by delivery model.

Despite the important contributions to the US health care system that nurse anesthetists have made for 150 years, and research evidence that validates their record of safety and cost-effectiveness, attempts by organized medicine to discredit the profession and restrict CRNA practice rights continue to the present day.

Educational Requirements for Becoming a CRNA: Today and Tomorrow

Since 1998, all nurse anesthetists have been required to complete a rigorous, focused course of graduate-level education resulting in a master's degree; many members of the profession have gone on to pursue doctorate degrees, including the PhD. In 2007, the AANA announced its support of doctoral education for entry into nurse anesthesia practice by 2025, propelling nurse anesthetists to yet another level of preparedness on behalf of the patients they serve.

As of January 2012, the requirements for an individual to become a CRNA and maintain that status include the following:

- A Bachelor of Science in Nursing (BSN) or other appropriate baccalaureate degree
- A current license as a registered nurse
- At least 1 year of experience as a registered nurse in an acute care setting
- Graduation with a minimum of a master's degree from an accredited nurse anesthesia educational program
- Pass the national certification examination following graduation
- In order to be recertified, CRNAs must obtain a minimum of 40 hours of approved continuing education every 2 years, document substantial anesthesia practice, maintain current state licensure, and certify that they have not developed any conditions that could adversely affect their ability to practice anesthesia.

Nurse anesthesia education builds on prior nursing education and experience. The minimum curriculum incorporates studies in basic and advanced applied sciences as well as principles and professional aspects of nurse anesthesia. Because these programs usually exist in colleges of nursing or allied health or schools of medicine, differing curricular requirements round out the course content based on the particular requirement of the department, school, or college in which they are located. Most programs require research, and many require completion of a project or thesis for graduation.

Nurse anesthesia educational programs are 24 to 36 months in length, and confer a master's degree on successful completion. These programs provide an educationally sound curriculum combining theory and clinical practice. Within the clinical component, each student is required to administer a minimum number of anesthetic agents to patients and work a minimum number of hours of anesthesia time. To meet these requirements, students provide the anesthesia services under the supervision of qualified clinical instructors, including CRNAs and/or anesthesiologists.

CRNAs are prepared to administer all types of anesthesia (general, regional, local, and conscious sedation), use all anesthesia and adjunctive drugs, determine need for and manage fluid and blood therapy, monitor and interpret data from sophisticated monitoring devices, insert invasive catheters (intravenous, central venous, and pulmonary artery catheters), recognize and correct complications that occur during the course of anesthesia, provide airway and ventilatory support, manage resuscitation efforts for cardiopulmonary arrest or serious injury, and provide pain management services.

Although the AANA had long discussed the possibility of nurse anesthesia education transitioning to the doctorate, the concept took on a different emphasis in 2004 when the American Association of Colleges of Nursing (AACN) published a position statement on the doctorate in nursing practice that addressed transformational change in the education required for entry into advanced nursing practice. Titled "Position Statement on the Practice Doctorate in Nursing," the AACN envisioned a practice doctorate requirement for all advanced practice nurses (APNs) for entry into practice by 2015. CRNAs were identified in the cadre of APNs.

Nurse anesthesia educational requirements have advanced significantly since Agatha Hodgins and her colleagues founded the AANA in 1931. Early on, the profession identified a primary objective to develop standards for nurse anesthesia education; over the years these standards for nurse anesthesia programs have evolved to meet the required knowledge and skills for entry into practice. In the 1980s, nurse anesthesia educational programs moved from hospital-based certificate programs to university-based graduate programs, and, in 1998, the Council on Accreditation of Nurse Anesthesia Educational Programs (COA) finalized the requirement that all programs award a master's or higher-level degree.

From the mid-1980s to the late 1990s, the AANA and the COA periodically assessed the need for, and feasibility of, practice-oriented doctoral degrees for nurse anesthetists. After the AACN adopted its position statement in October 2004, the AANA Board of Directors convened an invitational summit meeting of stakeholders in June 2005 to discuss interests and concerns surrounding doctoral preparation for nurse anesthetists. Pursuant to the summit meeting and with the approval of the Board of Directors, a Task Force on Doctoral Preparation of Nurse Anesthetists (DTF) was appointed. The DTF was charged with developing options relative to doctoral preparation of nurse anesthetists that the AANA Board could consider. To accomplish this, the task force held numerous meetings, conducted surveys, and held open hearings at AANA national meetings. The DTF's final report and options were presented to the board in April 2007. After much dialogue and debate, the AANA announced its support for doctoral education for entry into nurse anesthesia practice by 2025. The AANA Position on Doctoral Preparation of Nurse Anesthetists was announced to the membership in August 2007, with the following rationale for the decision presented:

- AANA has advanced quality education
- CRNAs are prepared safe providers
- To best position CRNAs to meet ongoing challenges and remain recognized anesthesia leaders.

When the AANA was founded more than 80 years ago, one of the basic tenets for organizing was so that the association would advance quality education as the means to ensure that nurse anesthetists are the best-prepared, safest anesthesia providers possible. With today's health care environment changing at an extraordinary rate, providers are required to keep pace by continually expanding their knowledge base and skill sets like never before. To best position CRNAs to meet this ongoing challenge and remain recognized leaders in anesthesia care, the AANA thinks it is essential to support doctoral education that encompasses technological and pharmaceutical advances, informatics, evidence-based practice, systems approaches to quality improvement, health care business models, teamwork, public relations, and other subjects that will shape the future for anesthesia professionals and their patients.

The COA was in agreement with the AANA, lending its endorsement to the association's position to require doctoral education for entry into nurse anesthesia practice by 2025. However, the decision did have opposition. Some in the CRNA community objected, arguing that education at the doctoral level for nurse anesthetists was unnecessary, and that the increased cost of education would result in decreasing applicants to nurse anesthesia educational programs and ultimately a decline in workforce numbers. The medical community objected to doctoral education for APNs in general, voicing the concern that these specialized nurses would misrepresent themselves to patients in clinical areas. As the debate escalated, clinical access for nurse anesthesia students became jeopardized at some sites, especially those heavily controlled by anesthesiologists. An additional difficulty in the transition to doctoral education in nurse anesthesia is that doctoral degree titles vary widely, from Doctorate of Nursing Practice (DNP) to Doctorate of Nurse Anesthesia Practice (DNAP), the result of approximately 50% of all nurse anesthesia educational programs not residing in colleges of nursing.

Despite APN doctorates continuing to provoke debate, particularly within the physician community, more and more nurse anesthesia educational programs are making the transition to doctoral curriculum, and practicing CRNAs are enrolling at doctoral programs in increasing numbers.

NURSE ANESTHESIA PRACTICE: WHAT THE FUTURE HOLDS

The AANA has been strengthened by and continues to flourish through the dedication of its members, volunteer leaders, and staff. This dedication will be critically important going forward, because, like all health care professionals, CRNAs are continually faced with managing change. Ongoing advancements in anesthesia technology, pharmacology, educational requirements, and practice standards have contributed significantly to anesthesia today being nearly 50 times safer than it was during the 1980s, regardless of provider type. Such changes for the good are easily managed compared with changes that may be perceived to have less favorable potential outcomes. A good example of the latter is the Obama administration's health reform plan with its attendant government wrangling, supply-and-demand economics, and rivalries between organized medicine and other health care professionals.

What does the future hold for nurse anesthesia? Although it is impossible to see very far into the future with any clarity, a clear picture of the near future becomes more visible by the day. Opportunities and challenges lie ahead in numerous areas, first and foremost technology, which keeps changing at a rapid pace. Few things highlight the differences between the generations like the ability and desire to keep up with, and adapt technology to, every facet of daily life. How might this affect health care professionals across generations working side by side in the clinical setting? Time will tell. In anesthesia, advancements to standard equipment such as anesthesia machines, monitors, laryngoscopes, and injection devices continue to improve the quality of patient care, keeping providers of all ages in a continual mode of learning and self-improvement and requiring practice standards and guidelines to be routinely reviewed and updated. In addition, technology is having a powerful impact on direct patient care as less invasive procedures are developed and used, leading to more outpatient procedures, shorter hospital stays, and faster patient recovery. The impact on nurse anesthesia has been, and will continue to be, a gradual migration of CRNAs from the traditional hospital setting to outpatient settings such as ambulatory surgery centers and physicians' offices. The development of robotic systems and artificial intelligence will also advance and the user interface for these seemingly futuristic tools will become simpler. Traditional ideas about safe practice will be tested as providers adapt the use of cell phones, iPads, laptops, and other mobile devices to clinical settings, including the operating room: What will ultimately be deemed acceptable and safe, and what will be considered taboo? Research evidence will ultimately frame the debates that occur and the decisions that get made.

In the education of student registered nurse anesthetists, the use of simulation will continue to develop as a means to impart and validate skills and knowledge without exposing patients to the process of clinical education; simulation will likely be used as part of the application process as well, to help identify and select candidates for admission to educational programs. Complex simulation will also play a larger role in the continuing education of certified providers, as Web-based modalities and other tools are used to deliver information and assess competency for practice.

Demonstration of health care provider competency will continue to be of paramount importance to patients, employers, insurers, lawmakers, and others with a vested interest in quality assurance. In nurse anesthesia, the movement to doctoral preparation and consideration of enhanced recertification requirements has sparked much discussion within the profession, but there is little doubt that education changes the world view, and as a body of doctorally prepared CRNAs emerges in the future, how the profession is perceived by its various publics will change for the better. CRNAs will be well prepared to take leadership positions on boards that shape health care systems, and to influence accountable care organizations, medical homes, and other entities yet to be envisioned.

Downward pressure on health care spending and changes in health care financing mechanisms intended to increase quality and care coordination while mitigating cost growth will shape CRNA practice and demand for CRNA services. New models of reimbursement and health care financing will be developed, with movement away from capitated payment to fee-for-service and volume-based payment to outcome-based payment systems. As these changes evolve, the type of practitioner providing care will become less important than the result of treatment, further eroding the artificially defined scope of practice boundaries. To lower costs, purchasers of health care services will seek lower-cost professionals and methods of care delivery, which in some circumstances will reduce, and in others increase, demand for CRNA services.

Increased interprofessional collaboration in health care will be expected, perhaps even mandated, because the US health system is rapidly reaching a point at which inefficient use of resources and duplication of efforts cannot be sustained and should not be tolerated. The Institute of Medicine's 2010 report on the "Future of Nursing" clearly identified that the United States needs to carefully consider how to make the best use of highly qualified APNs to drive a more efficient and effective health care system. Collaboration and cooperation across the broad spectrum of health care professionals and the organizations that represent them is essential.

How will CRNAs manage such change? With the same vigilance, preparation, determination, knowledge, experience, and ability that serve them so well caring for their patients every day. By continuing to provide patient access to safe, cost-effective anesthesia care; knowing the direction in which health care is headed; being politically active at the state and federal levels; educating the public about the value of nurse anesthetists; and being involved at the local community and institutional levels, CRNAs will continue to thrive today and in the future.

RESOURCES AND FURTHER READINGS

American Association of Nurse Anesthetists Archives, 222 South Prospect, Park Ridge (IL), 60068–4001.

Certified Registered Nurse Anesthetists (CRNAs) at a glance fact sheet. AANA, August 2011.

Quality of Care in Anesthesia. Park Ridge (IL): AANA; 2009.

Bankert M. Watchful care: a history of America's nurse anesthetists. New York: Continuum; 1989.

Thatcher VS. History of anesthesia with emphasis on the nurse specialist. Philadelphia: JB Lippincott; 1953.

Advancing the art and science of anesthesia for 75 years: a pictorial history of the American Association of Nurse Anesthetists. Park Ridge (IL): AANA; 2006.

The Doctorate in Nursing Practice
Moving Advanced Practice Nursing Even Closer to Excellence

Robin Donohoe Dennison, DNP, APRN, CCNS, CEN, CNE[a],*,
Camille Payne, PhD, RN[b], Kathleen Farrell, DNSc, BC, CCNS, ARNP[c]

KEYWORDS

- Advanced practice nurse • Doctor of nursing practice • Advanced degree
- Advanced practice registered nurse (APRN)

KEY POINTS

- The doctor of nursing practice (DNP) provides nursing with an opportunity to continue to define and strengthen clinical practice.
- The development of Advanced Practice Registered Nurses (APRNs) at the highest order of critical thinking and cognitive development in clinical practice and skills will serve to improve patient care and outcomes.
- Evolving issues should be visualized as challenges and opportunities to allow APRNs to have a greater impact on the healthcare system and patient outcomes.

One of the most significant events to affect advanced practice nursing is the practice doctorate. Controversial in its inception, the DNP is now firmly established as an educational path alternative to the traditional academic research doctoral degree. The DNP, as a practice doctorate, provides unique opportunities for nursing practice and education. APRNs can be empowered to achieve academic and credentialing parity with other health disciplines. Empowerment creates a needed paradigm shift from an academic focus on knowledge and skills in research methodologies to advancing knowledge and skills in the performance of practice as the essential core of nursing. Furthermore, the DNP expands available options for nurses who desire to advance their education. This article reviews the historical context that led to the introduction of the DNP and the proposal of the DNP as entry into practice for APRNs, DNP program parameters, and some of the evolving issues surrounding nursing's practice doctorate.

---

[a] Georgetown University, School of Nursing and Health Studies, 3700 Reservoir Road, Washington, DC 20057, USA
[b] Kennesaw State University, Kennesaw, GA, USA
[c] Murray State University, Murray, KY, USA
* Corresponding author.
E-mail address: rddennison@aol.com

Nurs Clin N Am 47 (2012) 225–240
doi:10.1016/j.cnur.2012.04.001
0029-6465/12/$ – see front matter © 2012 Elsevier Inc. All rights reserved.

nursing.theclinics.com

HISTORY

A historical review by Ivey[1] of the development of doctoral education in nursing notes that its foundations were in the doctor of education degree (EdD). The PhD was developed to prepare nurse researchers and nurse leaders needed by the profession. Statistics, research design, theory development, informatics, health policy, and outcomes measurement were emphasized. The development of doctoral programs in nursing then took divergent paths into the doctor of nursing (DNS), the doctor of nursing science (DNSc), the nursing doctor (ND), and the doctor of science in nursing (DSN). These degrees were developed within nursing programs, compared with PhD programs from graduate schools of universities, and were intended to be more clinically focused, hence more concerned with nursing issues and nursing practice. Curricula included nursing theory and strong research and statistics components and programs claimed to be either a clinical or a practice doctorate; however, on closer investigation, these programs offering DNSc, DNS, or DSN varied little from research doctoral programs. The American Association of Colleges of Nursing (AACN) Task Force on Quality Doctoral Education found few differences between curricula and requirements for PhD and DNS, DSN, and DNSc and recommended that the programs be designated research-focused doctorates.[2]

There are many reasons to add this educational opportunity for nurses. Starck and colleagues[3] predicted a shortage of clinically prepared leaders and called for an increase of doctoral-prepared faculty who would also be expert clinicians. Several recent publications from the Institute of Medicine have elucidated growing concerns about the safety of care, the quality of patient care delivery, and the achievement of health outcomes.[4–6] In a follow-up report, the Institute of Medicine stated, "all health professionals should be educated to deliver patient-centered care as members of an interdisciplinary team, emphasizing evidence-based practice, quality improvement approaches, and informatics."[7] The National Academy of Sciences[8] called for nursing to develop a practice doctorate to prepare expert clinicians. It stated, "The need for doctorally prepared practitioners and clinical faculty would be met if nursing could develop a new nonresearch clinical doctorate similar to the M.D. and Pharm.D. in medicine and pharmacy, respectively."[8] The increasing complexity of health care systems requires preparation at a higher level for APNs. Educational and clinical preparation at a doctoral level initiates and engages APNs at higher levels of clinical reasoning.

In 2002, a task force was convened by the AACN to assess the need for a nursing practice doctorate and clarify the purpose of such a doctoral degree. In 2004, the AACN issued a position statement calling for a transformational change in the education required for advanced nursing practice and for specialization in nursing to move from the master's level to the doctoral level.[9] The DNP was developed as a terminal degree and was intended to prepare graduates to provide the highest level of nursing practice. The AACN approved the DNP by October 2004. Several other health care professions, including pharmacy and physical therapy, have recently joined medicine and dentistry establishing practice doctorates as the entry level for their disciplines. The DNP is not designed for entry level into nursing, but it is a new entry into advanced nursing practice. Another reason for requiring a DNP for APNs is the achievement of parity with other doctoral-prepared health care professions. This positions the APN as a primary, important stakeholder at the political table for making health care decisions.

The DNP provides the advanced competencies required for increasingly complex clinical and leadership roles. The DNP competencies established by the AACN are described in *The Essentials of Doctoral Education for Advanced Nursing Practice*[10]

(**Table 1**). Conferring a doctoral degree for the time, program requirements, and credits for the education of APNs is a better match than a master's degree. Although most universities only require 30 semester hours for a master's degree, master's degree programs preparing graduates for APRN roles have continued to require more hours as the complexity of the role has increased so that credits at the master's level approached doctoral degree credit requirements without awarding a doctoral degree. Because APN master's degree programs average between 50 and 60 semester hours and are more hours than required for a master's degree in most other disciplines, it can be argued that the additional credits required to earn a DNP are a better value for the APN. In addition, professional students today expect to earn the higher degree recognition for an equivalent amount of time and other costs; therefore, nursing may lose quality prospective students to other disciplines if the terminal practice degree is not the entry point into advanced practice.

The AACN defines the term, *nursing practice*, broadly as referring to "any form of nursing intervention that influences health care outcomes for individuals or populations, including the direct care of individual patients, management of care for individuals or populations, administration of nursing and health care organizations, and the development and implementation of health policy."[10] A DNP is a degree, not a role. APRN roles include nurse anesthetist, nurse midwife, nurse practice, and clinical nurse specialist (CNS).

DNP EDUCATIONAL PROGRAMS

The AACN has proposed a dichotomy, with DNP the title for the practice-focused doctorate and PhD the title for the research-focused doctorate. Several programs, including those at Case Western Reserve University and University of Colorado, which offered practice doctorates with different titles (eg, ND) have converted their previous degrees to DNP whereas some programs that previously offered a DNSc, DNS, or DSN have converted their program titles to a either a DNP or PhD, depending on the focus of the program. Hathaway and colleagues[11] note that the pairing of professional and academic doctoral degrees within a discipline is common and gives the comparative examples of Doctor of Pharmacy (PharmD) and PhD in pharmacology, MD and PhD in a basic science, and EdD and PhD in education.

Nurses most likely to enroll in a DNP program are those who are committed to a career focusing on nursing practice and improving patient outcomes. These include APNs in direct delivery of care to individuals and populations, indirect delivery of care through a leadership role, and development and implementation of health policy.[12] The DNP is "expected to provide visionary leadership in nursing practice."[9]

The AACN has proposed a target date of 2015 for the preparation all new APNs to be at the doctoral level. Although not all schools of nursing will meet this target date, a new standard has been set and, as a result, institutions of higher learning around the country are developing DNP programs to meet the need. There are more than 184 DNP programs currently accepting students and more than 100 additional nursing schools are in the planning phase of offering DNP programs.[13] As the preparation of APNs moves from the master's level to the doctoral level, the need for DNP programs will continue to be in demand. Even though those nurses already licensed as APRNs will continue to be credentialed as such, many of these nurses can choose to complete their DNP though master of science in nursing (MSN) to DNP programs. APNs with a PhD may choose to also earn a DNP whereas nurses with a DNP may choose to also earn a PhD. Some schools are developing DNP/PhD programs in the vein of MD/PhD programs.

Table 1
The essentials of doctoral education for advanced nursing practice

Essential	Competency

Scientific underpinnings for practice	• Integrate nursing science with knowledge from ethics and the biophysical, psychosocial, analytical, and organizational sciences as the basis for the highest level of nursing practice
	• Use science-based theories and concepts to
	  ○ Determine the nature and significance of health and health care delivery phenomena
	  ○ Describe the actions and advanced strategies to enhance, alleviate, and ameliorate health and health care delivery phenomena as appropriate; and
	  ○ Evaluate outcomes
	• Develop and evaluate new practice approaches based on nursing theories and theories from other disciplines

Organizational and systems leadership for quality improvement and systems thinking	• Develop and evaluate care delivery approaches that meet current and future needs of patient populations based on scientific findings in nursing and other clinical sciences as well as organizational, political, and economic sciences
	• Ensure accountability for quality of health care and patient safety for populations with whom they work
	  ○ Use advanced communication skills/processes to lead quality-improvement and patient safety initiatives in health care systems
	  ○ Employ principles of business, finance, economics, and health policy to develop and implement effective plans for practice-level and/or system-wide practice initiatives that will improve the quality of care delivery
	  ○ Develop and/or monitor budgets for practice initiatives
	  ○ Analyze the cost-effectiveness of practice initiatives accounting for risk and improvement of health care outcomes
	  ○ Demonstrate sensitivity to diverse organizational cultures and populations, including patients and providers
	• Develop and/or evaluate effective strategies for managing the ethical dilemmas inherent in patient care, the health care organization, and research

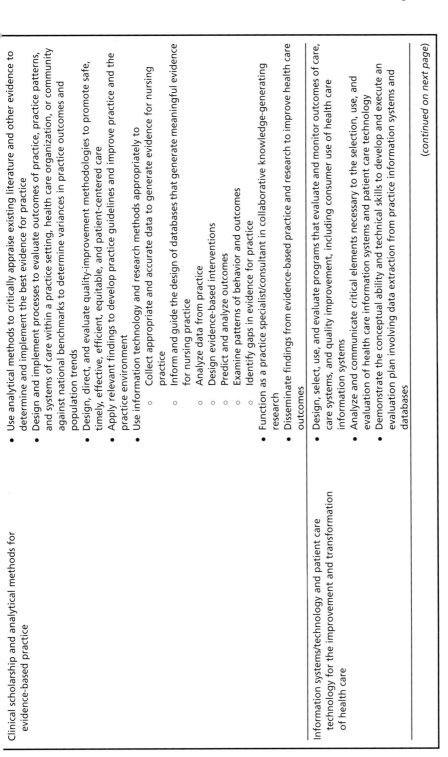

Clinical scholarship and analytical methods for evidence-based practice	• Use analytical methods to critically appraise existing literature and other evidence to determine and implement the best evidence for practice
	• Design and implement processes to evaluate outcomes of practice, practice patterns, and systems of care within a practice setting, health care organization, or community against national benchmarks to determine variances in practice outcomes and population trends
	• Design, direct, and evaluate quality-improvement methodologies to promote safe, timely, effective, efficient, equitable, and patient-centered care
	• Apply relevant findings to develop practice guidelines and improve practice and the practice environment
	• Use information technology and research methods appropriately to
	   ○ Collect appropriate and accurate data to generate evidence for nursing practice
	   ○ Inform and guide the design of databases that generate meaningful evidence for nursing practice
	   ○ Analyze data from practice
	   ○ Design evidence-based interventions
	   ○ Predict and analyze outcomes
	   ○ Examine patterns of behavior and outcomes
	   ○ Identify gaps in evidence for practice
	• Function as a practice specialist/consultant in collaborative knowledge-generating research
	• Disseminate findings from evidence-based practice and research to improve health care outcomes

Information systems/technology and patient care technology for the improvement and transformation of health care	• Design, select, use, and evaluate programs that evaluate and monitor outcomes of care, care systems, and quality improvement, including consumer use of health care information systems • Analyze and communicate critical elements necessary to the selection, use, and evaluation of health care information systems and patient care technology • Demonstrate the conceptual ability and technical skills to develop and execute an evaluation plan involving data extraction from practice information systems and databases

(continued on next page)

Table 1
(continued)

Essential	Competency
Health care policy for advocacy in health care	• Provide leadership in the evaluation and resolution of ethical and legal issues within health care systems relating to the use of information, information technology, communication networks, and patient care technology • Evaluate consumer health information sources for accuracy, timeliness, and appropriateness • Critically analyze health policy proposals, health policies, and related issues from the perspective of consumers, nursing, other health professions, and other stakeholders in policy and public forums • Demonstrate leadership in the development and implementation of institutional, local, state, federal, and/or international health policy • Influence policy makers through active participation on committees, boards, or task forces at the institutional, local, state, regional, national, and/or international levels to improve health care delivery and outcomes • Educate others, including policy makers at all levels, regarding nursing, health policy, and patient care outcomes • Advocate for the nursing profession within the policy and health care communities • Develop, evaluate, and provide leadership for health care policy that shapes health care financing, regulation, and delivery • Advocate for social justice, equity, and ethical policies within all health care arenas
Interprofessional collaboration for improving patient and population health outcomes	• Employ effective communication and collaborative skills in the development and implementation of practice models, peer review, practice guidelines, health policy, standards of care, and/or other scholarly products • Lead interprofessional teams in the analysis of complex practice and organizational issues • Employ consultative and leadership skills with intraprofessional and interprofessional teams to create change in health care and complex health care delivery systems
Clinical prevention and population health for improving the nation's health	• Analyze epidemiologic, biostatistical, environmental, and other appropriate scientific data related to individual, aggregate, and population health • Synthesize concepts, including psychosocial dimensions and cultural diversity, related to clinical prevention and population health in developing, implementing, and evaluating

	interventions to address health promotion/disease prevention efforts, improve health status/access patterns, and/or address gaps in care of individuals, aggregates, or populations • Evaluate care delivery models and/or strategies using concepts related to community, environmental and occupational health, and cultural and socioeconomic dimensions of health
Advanced nursing practice	• Conduct a comprehensive and systematic assessment of health and illness parameters in complex situations, incorporating diverse and culturally sensitive approaches • Design, implement, and evaluate therapeutic interventions based on nursing science and other sciences • Develop and sustain therapeutic relationships and partnerships with patients (individual, family, or group) and other professionals to facilitate optimal care and patient outcomes • Demonstrate advanced levels of clinical judgment, systems thinking, and accountability in designing, delivering, and evaluating evidence-based care to improve patient outcomes • Guide, mentor, and support other nurses to achieve excellence in nursing practice • Educate and guide individuals and groups through complex health and situational transitions • Use conceptual and analytical skills in evaluating the links among practice, organizational, population, fiscal, and policy issues

Data from The essentials of doctoral education for advanced nursing practice. American Association of Colleges of Nursing; 2006. Available at: http://www.aacn. nche.edu/dnp/Essentials.pdf.

DNP programs differ in whether they admit students with bachelor of science in nursing (BSN) degrees or students with MSN degrees (**Fig. 1**). MSN to DNP programs admit nurses who already have a master's degree and many of those programs require an APN credential for admission. These programs focus primarily on practice leadership and evidence-based practice and are usually approximately 40 semester credit hours. BSN to DNP programs admit nurses who have already earned BSNs and will complete their APN preparation during the DNP program. These programs are typically between 70 and 90 semester hours. Many universities that are offering BSN to DNP programs have eliminated the BSN to MSN option whereas others continue to offer the MSN option for APRN preparation.

Courses in the DNP programs are focused on the achievement of the competencies described in the AACN *Essentials* (**Fig. 2**; see **Table 1**). Typical courses include leadership, biostatistics, epidemiology, evidence-based practice, health care policy, finance and economics, quality improvement and outcomes management, and information technology.[14] BSN to DNP programs preparing graduates for an APRN role will have tracks specified by role and population. Most MSN to DNP programs do not have tracks but students select their areas of interest for their practica and terminal projects. Some MSN to DNP programs do have tracks; these most often focus on either direct or indirect care.[14]

All of these programs require practica, which are focused on the competencies as described in the AACN *Essentials*. As specified in the DNP Essential document, the Commission on Collegiate Nursing Education (CCNE) requires 1000 practicum hours post-BSN for the DNP. The BSN to DNP programs generally have 500-600 practicum hours focused on advanced practice with the remainder focused on practice leadership. Because most MSN programs preparing graduates for an APRN role require at

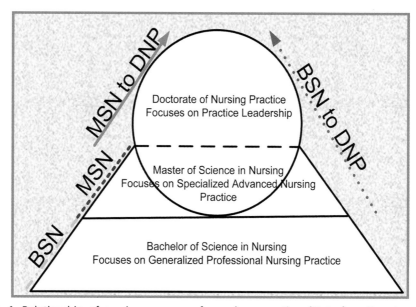

Fig. 1. Relationship of nursing programs focused on practice. (*Data from* Dennison RD. Second-generation DNP programs. Paper presented at the Sigma Theta Tau International Nursing Research Congress. Vancouver [Canada], 2009.)

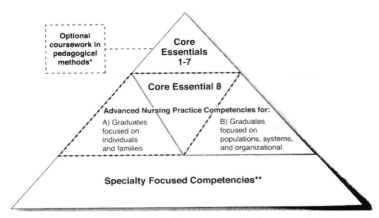

Fig. 2. Suggested DNP curriculum model. (*From* Moyer, Barbara Ann [2008]. *Nursing Education: Foundations for Practice Excellence* 1st edition, F.A. Davis Company, Philadelphia, PA; with permission.)

least 500 practicum hours, the MSN to DNP programs typically require 500 hours focused on practice leadership.

Most programs require some type of terminal project. The descriptions of these projects vary greatly but most focus on application of knowledge to improve practice and care outcomes. Although some schools have referred to these projects as a clinical dissertation or a thesis, the term capstone or scholarly project is preferred. Although there will be variation in quality, in general, the terminal project requires rigor. While the focus of the project is the implementation of research or other evidence into practice, the graduate also gains a better understanding of research is the consequential result, which can in turn improve research literacy benefiting students, peers, and practitioners in the evaluation of the evidence available for decision making.

Methodology of program delivery also varies. Some programs require students to attend courses on campus whereas other classes are online. Many are hybrid programs, however, delivered online but requiring on-campus attendance a few times per semester or immersion sessions with students coming to campus for a weekend, a week, or longer.

The CCNE is approving DNP programs using the AACN *Essentials* as the standard. The AACN AACN *Essentials* provides information regarding the evolution of the nursing practice doctorate as well as the placement and contextual position of the DNP into graduate nursing education. The AACN *Essentials* differentiates educational standards from master's-level advanced practice programs. Although the categories of essential statements are similar, a comparative review reveals higher levels of expectations for cognitive thinking and clinical practice.

The AACN *Essentials* provides an expectation for standards of quality. Although research doctoral programs do not participate in accreditation experiences, AACN (2010) has established criteria and standards for quality research-focused programs.[15] Also, literature surrounding doctoral programs is replete with articles describing quality indicators for graduate education. As early as 1982, Holzemer[16] published a key article on quality in graduate education, summarizing existing criteria in the literature and presenting a model for assessment of quality, which included standards, criteria, and indicators. More recently, Kim and colleagues[17] have discussed and summarized quality criteria, standards, and indicators for doctoral nursing programs across the globe. The AACN *Essentials* provides the framework for practice doctoral programs to establish measures of quality, ensuring some degree of consistency of education and performance for DNP graduates.

In a study by Loomis and colleagues,[18] the primary reasons that participants cited for deciding to pursue a DNP were increased intellectual knowledge and career advancement. Although more than half of the participants had considered pursuing a PhD, they chose a DNP over a PhD because they were not interested in a research-focused doctorate. The AACN offers an excellent comparison of the practice-focused and the research-focused doctorates to assist nurses with career decision making; it is available on their Web site (http://www.aacn.nche.edu/dnp/presentations/Grid8-05.pdf). The 2 types of doctoral degrees should be seen not as competitive but as complementary; the expectation is that DNPs and PhDs work collaboratively to advance nursing science and ensure the application of evidence-based practice to improve patient outcomes.[10]

More than half (55%) of the participants in Loomis and colleagues' study intended to work in nursing education after completing their DNP, whereas 39% planned to continue in clinical practice. The current shortage of nurses and nursing faculty is impeding the progress of expanding nursing educational programs to address practice shortages at all nursing levels. Predictions are that this faculty shortage will continue to rise significantly. With the rapid expansion of health care knowledge, nurses need more skills in knowledge use. Students can no longer be educated by having them simply memorize all content; rather, they must be provided the skills necessary to access and synthesize information, quickly using critical thinking and decision making to improve patient outcomes. Academic nursing programs need the advanced nursing knowledge, clinical expertise, and leadership of doctoral prepared faculty to prepare the next generation of nurses.

Doctoral education does not necessarily prepare graduates for teaching responsibilities even though many doctoral graduates in all disciples assume positions in academe. The AACN Position Statement on the DNP[9] states that the focus of the DNP should be on an advanced area of nursing practice. AACN does recommend that doctoral programs, both PhD or DNP, provide additional coursework or opportunities for individuals who may choose an academic career to attain these pedagogical skills. DNP programs are intended to prepare graduates at the highest level of nursing practice and focus on either direct care for individual patients or for indirect care eg, on systems, aggregates, policy or leadership in communities. Examples of the indirect care tracks may include administration, health policy, public health, and informatics. The DNP is a practice degree, not an education degree which is considered a separate discipline. However, the DNP, as is the PhD, is seen as an important preparation for faculty.

As DNP programs evolve, embedding preparation in pedagogy within the curriculum can be accomplished with creative curricular design and teaching strategies. Individual classes in instructional design, evaluation, and teaching and learning strategies are needed in both academic and practice settings. This content can be delivered in individually designed elective courses or integrated into didactic and practice activities and assignments.

Programs that include opportunities to select elective course encourage nurse educators or those aspiring to assume academic positions to use these electives to gain the skills necessary to assume such a role. Another approach may be to allow DNP students to serve as teaching assistants not only to aid in the development of the DNP students' practice knowledge and teaching skills but also as a contribution to the teaching mission of the schools, which occurs because undergraduate students benefit from the advanced clinical knowledge and practice skills of the DNP students.

EVOLVING ISSUES

Concerns about the DNP degree and especially about the DNP as a requirement for achievement of APRN status have been expressed. Many nurses claim that the MSN is sufficient, that APRNs are already experts, and that there is no need to mandate additional preparation. Research has shown that registered nurses with a BSN produce better patient outcomes than do registered nurses without a BSN.[19] It is, therefore, logical to expect that the new knowledge gained in a DNP program would have a significant impact on an APRN's practice and patient outcomes. The AACN DNP Essentials[10] were identified and then vetted by APRN and the nursing community at large as being essential for nurses practicing at this level in order to improve healthcare outcomes. As the profession pursues excellence for both nurses and patients, increasing educational expectations for APNs is a logical step in the process.

Although the DNP can be seen as positive because it provides parity for APRNs working side by side with other doctoral-prepared health care professionals, many healthcare providers claim that the nurse-doctor or doctor-nurse is confusing for patients. The term, *doctor*, is an academic title, all those who have earned that academic degree are authorized to use the title. MD, PhD, and DNP are degrees; physician and nurse are roles. In 2008, the American Medical Association proposed a resolution that opposed the use of the title "doctor" by nonphysicians but it was later modified to protect only the title "physician." Communication, establishing rapport, and developing trusting partnerships with patients and families are considered characteristic traits in which APRNs excel; therefore, APRNs are careful to identify and explain their role to patients and families, clarifying that they are advanced practice registered nurses.

Some healthcare providers claim that the additional time and money for achieving APRN preparation will actually contribute to a shortage of APRNs when there is an increasing demand. DNP preparation adds approximately 1 year to the typical MSN preparation for APRNs. Although a typical APN master's degree is approximately 45 to 50 semester credits, the post-BSN DNP is approximately 70 to 90 semester credits and adds to tuition costs. It is hoped that financial aid will be increasingly available to assist nurses in achieving this degree. Cronenwett and colleagues[20] cite multiple current events within nursing education and practice that will cause the 2015 target date for DNP entry into advanced practice to have a significant impact on the APRN workforce. They include the aging population, shortage of nursing faculty, health care reform, and economic challenges as factors that they indicate raise concerns regarding the 2015 target date.

Many nurses question the return on investment, especially if they are already APRNs and are approaching retirement. APRNs are not required to earn a DNP but are legally grandfathered to the APRN credential that they currently hold within the state that they practice. However, depending on how many additional earning years an individual has and personal career goals, he/she may choose to return to school to earn the DNP degree. Many APRNs argue that the DNP will not result in a higher salary, although that will be seen as more APRNs earn DNPs; employers do not generally raise salaries based solely on an employee's degrees.[12] Registered nurses with BSNs do not universally have a higher income than those with associate degrees, and APNs with a DNP will not universally have a higher income than those with a master's degree. Many factors influence salary levels, including position, role, geographic area, and demonstrated outcomes. In addition, the DNP may offer other employment opportunities for APRNs because they will have the necessary credentials to teach in various levels or types of nursing programs and the leadership skills sought by a variety of organizations and healthcare systems. The DNP will afford APRNs to be more marketable.

There are several questions related to faculty for the DNP programs. Because the same faculty members who now teach the APRN courses in master's programs would likely teach the advanced practice courses in DNP programs, the question of faculty workload is significant. This has led many programs to close their master's programs as they initiate their post-BSN DNP program. Another consideration is that many programs use MSN-prepared faculty to teach in their MSN programs. Although faculty members are encouraged to earn doctoral degrees, the use of faculty members with less than a doctoral degree in DNP programs is controversial. This controversy is in part a result of the lack of clear standards for faculty preparation. Neither the CCNE nor the National League for Nursing Accrediting Commission require graduate faculty to have doctorates. Although several of the higher education commissions also do not require doctorates for graduate faculty, the Southern Association of Colleges and Schools states specifically that faculty teaching graduate and postbaccalaureate course work have an earned doctorate/terminal degree in the teaching discipline or a related discipline.[21] The AACN DNP Essentials[10] states that Master's prepared faculty members may be the best to teach particularly the clinical courses in the DNP program during the transition.

Many new DNP programs are starting their programs with several faculty members in their first classes and some with the entire first class composed of faculty members from within the school. This "grow your own" philosophy is difficult for faculty colleagues either as course faculty or students and introduces a potential conflict of interest. Anselmi and colleagues[22] explored the faculty as student issue from the perspectives of faculty member, department chair, associate dean, and dean. They provide recommendations for limiting conflict of interest and maintaining quality of rigor of the doctoral education while optimizing the opportunities for facilitating doctoral education for faculty members. These include policy statements regarding faculty members who are students in their own school and college and faculty exchange programs so that faculty can attend another equivalent program. In addition, the effect of the relationship between student and a student who is also a faculty member needs to be explored. Camaraderie, trust, and teamwork among doctoral students are essential factors to consider.

A significant number of institutions that offer advanced practice degrees at the master's level are not approved for doctoral programs. As a solution to this problem, some of these programs have been able to receive approval from higher education administration at state or regional levels to offer practice doctorates only (EdD, Doctor of Physical Therapy (DPT), DNP, and so forth). Others have established joint programs with doctoral-granting institutions.

Some nurse leaders have argued that DNP programs will divert potential nurse scientists from PhD programs. Edwardson[23] asserts, "this is a real concern only if schools of nursing fail to insist on comparable rigor of the two programs."[(p138)] As previously stated, the rigor of the 2 types of doctoral programs should be the same but with a different the focus. In actuality, enrollment in DNP and PhD programs has increased since the advent of DNP programs.[24] Many nurses who wanted a doctoral degree but were not interested in a research-focused doctoral program chose not to enroll in a doctoral program when a practice-focused option was not available. Other nurses earned a PhD because they had embarked on an academic career and were advised to earn a terminal degree but never intended to develop a program of research. Because only 1% of US nurses hold a doctoral degree,[24] having a practice doctorate option available will allow nurses who are interested in earning a doctoral degree to make wise career choices. The Institute of Medicine report, *The Future of Nursing*, recommends doubling the number of nurses with a doctorate by 2020[25]; having a doctoral degree with a practice focus increases the pool of potential nursing doctoral candidates.

Academicians frequently call for the DNP capstone projects to have the same rigor as a dissertation. Unlike a dissertation, the terminal project in a DNP program is intended to be a culmination experience with application of evidence rather than generation of new knowledge. DNP students are expected to complete 1000 practicum hours refining their practice leadership rather than the hours that PhD students spend on the dissertation process and engaged in conducting research. Hathaway and colleagues[11] claim that the distinction between professional and academic degrees is not one of rigor but rather focus of study. The DNP's focus of study is on practice, application of existing evidence, and improvement of health care outcomes.

There are many questions about the DNP in academe. Hathaway and colleagues[11] claim that the DNP programs offer greater prospect to ease the faculty shortage than do research-focused PhD programs. A DNP in a faculty role will devote more time to teaching than a PhD, whose focus is on developing a program of research and whose teaching workload is likely to be approximately half the credit hours as a DNP in a teaching or practice track. Edwardson[23] writes that the relative proportion of PhD and DNP faculty should be dictated by a school's mission. She goes on to say that if research is the key mission of the school, there would logically be a higher number of PhD-prepared faculty members but these schools would benefit from having DNP-prepared faculty members to fulfill the teaching and service missions. In schools that have a primary teaching mission, especially with a heavy APN focus, there would logically be more clinically current DNP-prepared faculty members.

Even though the DNP is considered a terminal degree, some schools or colleges do not consider nurses without a PhD for tenure track positions whereas others offer the tenure-track option to nurses with a DNP. Because earning tenure is different from being eligible for tenure, the reappointment, promotion, and tenure criteria and the schools' definitions of scholarship must be considered. If the criteria include research and external funding for research, it is likely that a DNP would have difficulty meeting criteria for tenure. Research-track faculty must be focused on research, teaching, and service in that order; teaching or clinical track faculty are going to be more focused on teaching and practice with requirements for clinical scholarship and service. DNP faculty members are qualified to teach clinical practice in undergraduate programs and advanced practice in graduate programs as well as leadership, health policy, and evidence-based practice in undergraduate or graduate programs. Some schools and colleges have implemented or are considering parallel tenure tracks, one focused on teaching and/or practice and the other focused on research.

RESPONSES OF APRN PROFESSIONAL ASSOCIATIONS

APRNs are represented by several professional organizations. Membership of the American Nurses Association and the National League for Nursing includes nurses of all specialties and educational levels, whereas numerous APRN organizations exist for the support and advancement of APRN roles and specialties. Organizations representing the 4 APRN roles have issued current positions on the DNP initiative.[26]

Nurse Anesthesia

The American Association of Nurse Anesthetists (AANA) has mandated that all certified registered nurse anesthetist (CRNA) programs transition to a practice doctorate by 2022 and that by 2025, all new CRNA graduates must hold a practice doctorate to be eligible for certification.[27] Also, the AANA Council on Accreditation will not accredit new master's degree programs for nurse anesthesia after 2015.[24]

Nurse Midwifery

The American College of Nurse-Midwives currently endorses the master's degree as basic preparation for midwifery practice but does support a variety of doctoral degree options for midwifery programs. Although they recognize the DNP as an option for midwifery programs, they are not mandating a DNP requirement for certification as a nurse midwife or that midwifery programs be converted to DNP programs. They do recognize the need to develop competencies for midwifery education at the doctoral level.[28]

Nurse Practitioners

Seven nurse practitioner organizations comprise the Nurse Practitioner Roundtable for the purposes of addressing nurse practitioner issues, collaborating efforts, and presenting a unified position on policy and legislative efforts. All 7 of the nurse practitioner organizations (ie, American Academy of Nurse Practitioners, American College of Nurse Practitioners, Association of Faculties of Pediatric Nurse Practitioners, National Association of Nurse Practitioners in Women's Health, National Association of Pediatric Nurse Practitioners , National Conference of Gerontological Nurse Practitioners, and the National Organization of Nurse Practitioner Faculties) have issued a statement indicating that the DNP reflects current clinical competencies and prepares the nurse practitioner for the changing health care system.[29] NONPF approved new core nurse practitioner competencies in 2011; these are at a doctoral level (NONPF, 2012).[30]

Clinical Nurse Specialists

Although the National Association of Clinical Nurse Specialists (NACNS) has maintained a neutral position on the DNP, the organization supports CNS education at a master's level or doctoral level.[31] Although NACNS does not support the elimination of MSN programs to move to the DNP as entry into CNS practice, the NACNS Board of Directors directed the development of doctoral-level CNS competencies, which have now been completed, posted, and endorsed by several other organizations.[31] The Society for Clinical Nurse Specialists Education has endorsed the DNP and is developing curriculum guidelines for CNS tracks within DNP programs (C. Payne, PhD, RN, personal communication, March 29, 2012).

SUMMARY

Although it is likely that the DNP will remain controversial for the next decade, it is also evident that this degree has been ardently embraced by individual nurses seeking advanced degrees that focus on nursing practice and by the nursing community itself. Each of the 4 APRN roles has developed task forces or committees to explore entry into advanced practice at the DNP level. As APRNs continue to seek and develop consensus regarding the nature and experience of advanced practice nursing, the nursing practice doctorate will concurrently continue to grow and mature. The DNP provides nursing with a singular opportunity to continue to define and strengthen clinical practice. The development of APNs at the highest order of critical thinking and cognitive development in clinical practice and skills will serve not only to vitalize nursing but also to improve patient care and outcomes in ways not yet defined, given the infancy of the DNP. Controversies and concerns should be visualized as critical challenges to overcome flaws and impediments in existing educational structures and processes. The DNP should be the opportunity that unites advanced practice nursing, exemplifies clinical practice, and defines the very nature of nursing.

REFERENCES

1. Ivey J. The preparation of nurse faculty: who should teach students. Top Adv Pract Nurs 2007;7:2. Available at: http://www.medscape.com/viewarticle/561575. Accessed March 29, 2012.
2. Author. Position statement on quality indicators for doctoral programs. Washington, DC: American Association of Colleges of Nursing; 2001.
3. Starck PL, Duffy ME, Vogler R. Developing a nursing doctorate for the 21st century. J Prof Nurs 1993;9(4):212–9.
4. Aspden P, Corrigan JM, Wolcott J, et al, editors. Patient safety. Achieving a new standard for care. Washington, DC: The National Academies Press; 2004.
5. Institute of Medicine. Crossing the quality chasm. A new health system for the 21st century. Washington, DC: National Academy Press; 2001.
6. Kohn LT, Corrigan JM, Donaldson MS, editors. To err is human. Building a safer health system. Washington, DC: National Academy Press; 2000.
7. Greiner AC, Knebel E, editors. Health professions education: a bridge to quality. Washington, DC: Institute of Medicine of the National Academies; 2003. p. 3.
8. National Academy of Sciences. Advancing the nation's health care needs: NIH research training programs. Washington, DC: National Academies Press; 2005. p. 74.
9. AACN position statement on the practice doctorate in nursing. American Association of Colleges of Nursing; 2004. p. 10; second citation. Available at: http://www.aacn.nche.edu/DNP/DNPPositionStatement.htm. Accessed March 28, 2012.
10. The essentials of doctoral education for advanced nursing practice. American Association of Colleges of Nursing; 2006. Available at: http://www.aacn.nche.edu/dnp/Essentials.pdf. Accessed March 28, 2012.
11. Hathaway D, Jacob S, Stegbauer C, et al. The practice doctorate: perspectives of early adopters. J Nurs Educ 2006;45(12):487–96.
12. Clinton P, Sperhac AM. National agenda for advanced practice nursing: the practice doctorate. J Prof Nurs 2006;22(1):7–14.
13. DNP program schools. American Association of Colleges of Nursing; 2012. Available at: http://www.aacn.nche.edu/dnp/program-schools. Accessed March 28, 2012.
14. Dennison RD. Second-generation DNP programs. Paper presented at the Sigma Theta Tau International Nursing Research Congress. Vancouver (Canada), July 14, 2009.
15. American Association of Colleges of Nursing. 2010. The Research-focused doctoral program in nursing. Pathways to excellence. Available at: www.aacn.nche.edu/education-resources/phdposition.pdf. Accessed April 16, 2012.
16. Holzemer WL. Quality in graduate nursing education. Nurs Health Care 1982;3(10):536–42.
17. Kim MJ, McKenna HP, Ketefian S. Global quality criteria, standards, and indicators for doctoral programs in nursing; literature review and guideline development. Int J Nurs Stud 2006;43:477–89.
18. Loomis JA, Willard B, Cohen J. Difficult professional choices: deciding between the PhD and the DNP in nursing. Online J Issues Nurs 2006;12(1):6.

19. Aiken LH, Clarke SP, Cheung RB, et al. Educational levels of hospital nurses and surgical patient mortality. JAMA 2003;290(12):1617–23.

20. Cronenwett L, Dracup K, Grey M, et al. The doctor of nursing practice: a national workforce perspective. Nurs Outlook 2011;59(1):9–17.

21. The principles of accreditation: foundations for quality enhancement. Author. Decatur (GA): Southern Association of Colleges and Schools Commission on Colleges; 2012.

22. Anselmi KK, Dreher HM, Glasgow ME, et al. Faculty colleagues in your classroom as doctoral students: is there a conflict of interest? Nurse Educ 2010; 35(5):213–9.

23. Edwardson S. Doctor of philosophy and doctor of nursing practice as complementary degrees. J Prof Nurs 2010;26(3):137–40.

24. Raines CF. The doctor of nursing practice: a report on progress. Paper presented at the American Association of Colleges of Nursing Spring Annual Meeting. Washington, DC, March 21, 2010.

25. The future of nursing: leading change, advancing health. Institute of Medicine; 2010. Available at: http://www.iom.edu/Reports/2010/The-Future-of-Nursing-Leading-Change-Advancing-Health.aspx. Accessed March 30, 2012.

26. Rhodes MK. Using effects-based reasoning to examine the DNP as the single entry degree for advanced practice nursing. Online J Issues Nurs 2011;16(3):8 American Nurses Association (ANA) at Available at: http://www.nursingworld.org/MainMenuCategories/ANAMarketplace/ANAPeriodicals/OJIN/TableofContents/Vol-16-2011/No3-Sept-2011. Accessed March 29, 2012.

27. AANA position on doctoral preparation of nurse anesthetists. American Association of Nurse Anesthetists; 2007. Available at: http://www.aana.com/ceandeducation/educationalresources/Documents/AANA_Position_DTF_June_2007.pdf. Accessed March 30, 2012.

28. Midwifery education and the doctor of nursing practice (DNP) position statement. American College of Nurse-Midwives; 2011. Available at: http://www.midwife.org/ACNM/files/ACNMLibraryData/IPLAODFILENAME/000000000079/Midwifery%20Ed%20and%20DNP%207.09.pdf. Accessed March 29, 2012.

29. Nurse Practitioner Roundtable. (2008). Nurse practitioner DNP education, certification and titling: a unified statement. Available at: http://www.afpnp.org/DNPUnifiedStatement0608.pdf. Accessed March 29, 2012.

30. National Organization of Nurse Practitioner Faculties. 2012. Competencies for nurse practitioners. Available at: http://www.nonpf.com/displaycommon.cfm?an=1&subarticlenbr=14. Accessed April 16, 2012.

31. National Association of Clinical Nurse Specialists. White paper on the nursing practice doctorate 2009. Available at: http://www.nacns.org/docs/PositionOnNursingPracticeDoctorate.pdf. Accessed March 29, 2012.

Impact of New Regulatory Standards on Advanced Practice Registered Nursing
The APRN Consensus Model and LACE

Joan M. Stanley, PhD, RN, CRNP

KEYWORDS

• APRN regulation • Consensus model • Nursing leadership

KEY POINTS

• As health care needs increase, the advanced practice registered nurse (APRN) is an effective part of meeting those needs.
• The Consensus Model for APRN Regulation provides a framework to increase the APRN's role and improve health outcomes in the United States.
• The goal of implementation of the Consensus Model by 2015 will require a unified effort by the nursing profession to meet health care needs.

The challenges facing the United States health care system are real and unsettling. The nation's population is aging rapidly, with more than 20% of the population expected to be 65 years and older by 2030.[1] We are bombarded with reports that rates of chronic diseases in children and adults are increasing at alarming rates. Despite having the highest per capita expenditure for health care in the world,[2] the United States ranks 30th in infant mortality rates[3] and ranks last out of 16 countries in preventable deaths.[4] These figures are only a sampling of data that constantly remind us of the urgent need to increase access to quality health care services, and rethink the type and way that care is delivered in the current health care system.

Workforce projections show that more than 150,000 additional physicians will be needed in the next 10 to 15 years to meet the goal of providing health care access to all United States citizens (Association of American Medical Colleges, 2009). This shortage is expected to be even more acute for physicians prepared to provide primary care services. According to the American Academy of Family Physicians, the United States will need 40% more primary care providers by 2020 to meet the nation's demand

American Association of Colleges of Nursing One Dupont Circle, NW, Suite 530, Washington, DC 20036, USA
E-mail address: jstanley@aacn.nche.edu

doi:10.1016/j.cnur.2012.02.001
0029-6465/12/$ – see front matter © 2012 Elsevier Inc. All rights reserved.
nursing.theclinics.com

for primary care services. This concern is magnified by the fact that only 2% of all new physicians opted for primary care or general medicine residencies in 2008.[5]

One promising and effective way to bridge the gap between needed and available primary care providers is to increase the production of Advanced Practice Registered Nurses (APRNs), particularly of nurse practitioners (NPs) and clinical nurse specialists (CNSs). APRNs are increasingly used to fill gaps in care, and represent a significant component of the United States health care workforce and providers of primary care services. A Government Accounting Office[6] report on primary care projections and trends showed that NPs are the fastest growing group of primary care providers in the country. APRNs also have repeatedly been shown to provide high-quality care, typically at a lower cost.[7–11]

According to the 2008 National Sample Survey of Registered Nurses,[12,13] an estimated 250,527 or 8.2% of registered nurses were prepared as APRNs, an increase from an estimated 240,460 in 2004. This estimate, however, may not tell the full story. The lack of common titling, regulatory requirements, and recognition across states hinder the ability to accurately identify the number of APRNs practicing in the United States. Also, the numbers of APRNs may be higher than estimated because they have been historically billed under a physician's name or as part of hospital services and are not counted separately in federal databases.

Despite the lack of definitive numbers, APRNs represent a significant and crucial resource to meeting the country's growing health care needs. However, these resources must be used to the full extent and in the most effective way possible. The Institute of Medicine (IOM) report, *Future of Nursing: Leading Change, Advancing Health*, recognizes the importance of APRNs in meeting the country's health care needs and delineates 4 key messages that directly affect advanced practice registered nursing.

1. Nurses should practice to the full extent of their education and training.
2. Nurses should achieve higher levels of education and training through an improved education system that promotes seamless academic profession.
3. Nurses should be full partners, with physicians and other health professionals, in redesigning health care in the United States.
4. Effective workforce planning and policy making require better data collection and an improved information infrastructure.[14(p4)]

The advanced practice nursing community, through the development of the Consensus Model for APRN Regulation: Licensure, Accreditation, Certification and Education (LACE),[15] has positioned itself to assume a leadership role within the health care system and participate as an equal partner in redesigning health care in the United States. The Consensus Model, reprinted in the appendix of the IOM report, has been recognized by policy makers and others outside of nursing as foundational to the future of APRN practice. Implementation, although still relatively early in the process, will be even more critical as nursing moves toward achieving this goal. Ongoing, transparent communication among all LACE entities has been recognized as the most critical component in achieving and maintaining consensus as advanced practice nursing moves toward the goal of full implementation of this new regulatory model by 2015.

In early 2004, after repeatedly hearing reports that CNSs and NPs were not able to be certified or licensed to practice after graduating from an APRN program or that APRNs moving to another state were no longer able to practice, the American Association of Colleges of Nursing (AACN) and the National Organization of Nurse

Practitioner Faculties (NONPF) jointly presented their concerns to the Alliance for APRN Credentialing (the Alliance). The Alliance, created in 1997, was convened by the AACN to provide a forum to regularly discuss issues related to nursing education, practice, and credentialing. The membership comprises organizations that accredit APRN programs, certify APRNs, and develop APRN educational standards. The Alliance agreed to convene a national consensus process and invited 50 organizations to participate. The first APRN Consensus Conference was held June 2004 and included representatives of 32 organizations focused on APRN practice, education, certification, accreditation, or licensure. Barbara Safriet, an attorney and long-time advocate for APRN full scope of practice, chaired this first consensus conference, which ultimately led to the development of what has become known as the Consensus Model, which delineates the future model for all APRN regulation.

As an outcome of the first consensus conference, the Alliance formed a workgroup comprising representatives from 23 organizations, and charged them with developing a consensus statement that addresses the issues that had been identified with the goal of creating a future model for APRN regulation. Jean Johnson, Senior Associate Dean for Health Sciences at George Washington University and a gerontology NP, was asked to facilitate this consensus process, which eventually extended over a 5-year period. As the APRN Work Group was beginning its work, the American Nurses Association (ANA), in collaboration with the AACN, convened a second stakeholders' meeting in December 2004. This meeting reinforced the need to address the multitude of issues surrounding APRN regulation. Over the next several years, participation in this larger consensus process grew to more than 60 nursing organizations that self-identified as having a stake in APRN regulation. The AACN and ANA reconvened the larger APRN stakeholder group several times throughout the 5-year consensus building process to share and solicit feedback on recommendations as they emerged. In 2006, the National Council of State Boards of Nursing (NCSBN) APRN Advisory Panel, having drafted its own report on APRN regulation, met with the APRN Work Group to discuss areas of common agreement and disagreement. As discussions continued, both groups agreed that one joint report should be developed that addressed the future regulation of advanced practice nursing. In 2008, the Consensus Model for APRN Regulation: Licensure, Accreditation, Certification and Education was finalized by the APRN Joint Dialogue Group (comprising representatives of the NCSBN APRN Advisory Panel and the APRN Consensus Work Group) and was disseminated widely. Forty-eight nursing organizations quickly endorsed the Model and implementation began immediately. The complete list of endorsing organizations and those participating in the APRN Work Group, the APRN Joint Dialogue Group, and the larger consensus process can be found in the document at http://www.aprnlace. org. Because the Model has significant implications for all APRN regulation and practice, every APRN is strongly encouraged to access and read the entire document and to stay up to date regarding ongoing decisions and processes as implementation continues over the next several years.

LACE AND IMPLEMENTATION OF THE CONSENSUS MODEL

The Consensus Model report recommended the creation of a formal communication mechanism known as LACE, which includes those regulatory organizations that represent APRN licensure, accreditation, certification, and education entities. The purpose of LACE is to provide a formal mechanism for facilitating transparent and aligned communication among all stakeholders. In 2010, 28 organizations signed an agreement to support the creation and maintenance of this electronic platform. LACE, not a separate or formal organization, provides a mechanism to communicate current information regarding the implementation of the Consensus Model to the public and provides a platform for APRN regulatory bodies to share updates regarding implementation, discuss concerns that arise, and work on joint positions or documents as needed. The LACE site can be accessed at http://www.aprnlace.org.

THE CONSENSUS MODEL: IMPLICATIONS FOR ALL APRNs

The Consensus Model delineates a model for the regulation of all APRNs and, therefore, has implications for all APRNs. Building on the model of regulation described by Styles,[16] the Model addresses the licensure, accreditation, certification, and education of all APRNs. Synergistic expectations and requirements for each of these regulatory components are delineated. The diagram depicting the APRN regulatory model is shown in **Fig. 1**.

Definition and Titling of an APRN

Advanced Practice Registered Nurse or APRN is the legal title used to recognize 4 distinct roles: certified registered nurse anesthetist (CRNA), certified nurse-midwife (CNM), CNS, and certified NP; and is the credential to be used by individuals licensed in any of these 4 roles. The definition of an APRN includes graduate-level education in 1 of the 4 recognized roles; national certification; preparation for health promotion as well as the assessment, diagnosis, and management of patient problems, which includes the use and prescription of pharmacologic and nonpharmacologic interventions; and the provision of direct care to patients.

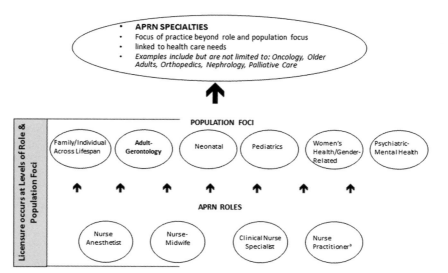

Fig. 1. The APRN Regulatory Model. [a] The Nurse Practitioner role is divided into acute care and primary care roles for the adult-gerontology and pediatric populations. (*From* APRN Consensus Work Group, & National Council of State Boards of Nursing APRN Advisory Committee. (2008). Consensus model for APRN regulation: licensure, accreditation, certification & education. Available at: http://www.aacn.nche.edu/education- resources/APRNReport.pdf. Accessed November 28, 2011.)

This definition provides clear parameters for APRNs. Only individuals who have graduated from an accredited APRN education program, are nationally certified, and are licensed under the criteria delineated in the Model may use the title APRN. The importance of other advanced areas of nursing practice that do not provide direct care to individuals, such as public health nursing, administration, and informatics, are recognized but not included in the definition of APRN.

Education

The Model stipulates that all APRNs must be educated in a graduate or postgraduate certificate program that prepares them in 1 of the 4 APRN roles and in at least 1 of 6 identified populations: across the life span/family, adult-gerontology, pediatrics, women's health/gender specific, psychiatric/mental health, and neonatal. The education must be broad and comprehensive in nature, and must prepare the graduate with the nationally recognized APRN core, role, and population-focused competencies. The program must ensure that graduates are eligible for national certification and state licensure, and the transcript or official documentation must specify the role and population focus of the graduate. Any specialty preparation in a more in-depth area of practice, such as in oncology, palliative care, or dermatology, may be included as part of the graduate education program or in a separate program, but must be over and above the broad comprehensive education in the role and population. The model for building the APRN curriculum is shown in **Fig. 2**.

One component of the Model that has caused some confusion is the bifurcation of the NP role. Under the Model, NPs prepared to provide care to the adult-gerontology or pediatric populations can be educated as either primary care NPs or acute care NPs, which have separate national consensus-based competencies and separate certification processes. Education programs may prepare graduates across both roles; however, graduates must be prepared with the competencies for both roles and must successfully obtain certification in both the acute and primary care NP roles.

Although not a new requirement, all APRN education must include the APRN core: 3 separate, graduate, comprehensive courses, commonly referred to as the 3 Ps: advanced health assessment, advanced physiology/pathophysiology, and advanced

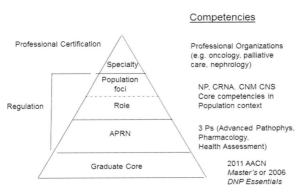

Competencies

Professional Certification

Professional Organizations
(e.g. oncology, palliative
care, nephrology)

Specialty

Population foci

NP, CRNA, CNM CNS
Core competencies in
Population context

Regulation   Role

APRN

3 Ps (Advanced Pathophys,
Pharmacology,
Health Assessment)

Graduate Core

2011 AACN
Master's or 2006
DNP Essentials

Fig. 2. Building an APRN curriculum. (*From* APRN Consensus Work Group, & National Council of State Boards of Nursing APRN Advisory Committee. (2008). Consensus model for APRN regulation: licensure, accreditation, certification & education. Available at: http://www. aacn.nche.edu/education- resources/APRNReport.pdf. Accessed November 28, 2011.)

pharmacology. The specific requirements for these 3 graduate-level APRN core courses are:

- Advanced health assessment must include all body systems and advanced techniques
- Advanced physiology/pathophysiology must include concepts across the entire life span, which is defined as prenatal through death, including the frail elderly
- Advanced pharmacology must include all broad categories of pharmacologic agents and not just those commonly used by the role/population.[15(p11)]

One commonly asked question regarding the APRN core is: can these 3 courses be designed for just one role or specific population, such as for pediatric NPs? Agreement among the LACE organizations clarifies that it is not who is sitting in the classroom, but rather the content and outcomes of the courses that are important. Therefore, if a course for pediatric NPs or any single APRN role or population is included in the program of study, the course content must meet the requirements as defined above. A clarifying statement on the 3 APRN core courses is posted on the LACE site at http://www.aprnlace.org. In addition to these 3 separate courses, additional content in these 3 areas must be included in the diagnostic and management courses specific to the role and population.

The 6 population-focused areas of practice present significant changes to the way APRNs, particularly NPs and CNSs, are educated and certified. The adult-gerontology population requires the merging of the current adult and gerontology curricula. Under this model, all NPs and CNSs prepared to care for the adult or gerontology populations must now be prepared with the competencies previously recognized for adult and gerontology practice. New national consensus-based competencies have been developed for the:

- Adult-gerontology acute care NP
- Adult-gerontology primary care NP
- Adult-gerontology CNS.

These competencies can be accessed at http://www.aacn.nche.edu/education-resources/competencies-older-adults. In addition to the redesign of the adult-gerontology APRN curriculum, these competencies are being used as a foundation for the development of new certification examinations for these 3 roles/population-focused areas of practice.

In addition to expanding the education of adult and gerontology NPs and CNSs, the Model recognizes the urgent need to prepare APRNs to care for the growing older adult population. Therefore, all APRNs who provide care to older adults, including the CRNA, CNM, women's health NP, psychiatric/mental health (psych/MH) NP, family NP, and women's health CNS, must have additional preparation in the care of the older adult. To facilitate these curricular modifications, recommended competencies for NPs and CNSs who care for older adults have been developed and can be found at http://www.aacn.nche.edu/education-resources/competencies-older-adults.

The Model also has significant implications for psychiatric/mental health APRNs. Under the Model, all psych/MH APRNs must be prepared across the life span. To examine the implications for psychiatric nursing and the changes that would need to be made to align psychiatric/mental health advanced practice nursing with the Model, the American Psychiatric Nurses Association and the International Society of Psychiatric Nurses appointed a joint task force. After extensive dialogue the task force made a series of recommendations, which have been adopted by both organizations, including that there be one entry educational focus: psychiatric/mental health NP with

preparation across the life span. Additional information regarding all recommendations can be accessed at http://www.apna.org/i4a/pages/index.cfm?pageid=4387.
Previous job analyses had shown little differentiation between the psych/MH NP
and CNS roles and practice. These 2 organizations continue to work with the other
education organizations to develop competencies for the psych/MH NP prepared to
provide care across the life span, and with certifiers to develop a new certification
examination for the role and across the life-span population. The impact on practice
and the potential need for additional specialty certification is also being discussed.

The inclusion of health maintenance and health promotion as a component of all
APRN education is also a new requirement and one that the certifying organizations
are concerned may be overlooked by APRN faculty. The health promotion/health maintenance content will vary depending on the role and population, but must be included in
the curriculum.

Accreditation

Under the Consensus Model, all APRN education programs must be accredited by
a national nursing or nursing-related accrediting body recognized by the Department
of Education or the Council for Higher Education Accreditation. This category includes
all graduate and postgraduate certificate programs. Another significant change is the
requirement that all new APRN programs or tracks must be preapproved or preaccre-
dited before students are admitted. Both the Commission on Collegiate Nursing
Education (CCNE) and the National League for Nursing Accrediting Commission
(NLNAC) have indicated that processes to carry out these new requirements will be
in place and fully implemented by 2012/2013.

Under the new regulatory model, the APRN accrediting bodies, which include the
CCNE, NLNAC, Council on Accreditation of Nurse Anesthesia Educational Programs
(COA), and Accreditation Commission for Midwifery Education (ACME), are also
charged with assuring that the education program includes the APRN core, role core,
and population core competencies. Graduates of these APRN education programs
must be eligible to sit for national certification in the role and population focus.

Certification

When the Consensus Model was finalized in 2008 several states, including some with
the largest number of APRNs, did not require national certification. Under the Model,
all APRNs must be nationally certified by an entity that is accredited by a national certification accrediting body. The certification examination must assess the APRN core,
role, and population-focused competencies. If a specialty is tested, it must be done
separately from the role and population.

All APRN certification organizations are assessing current examinations to determine
what changes are needed to meet the requirements of the Model. Some of these
changes include assessment of health promotion/health maintenance in all APRN certification examinations, and an emphasis on care of the older adult for all APRNs
prepared to provide care to adults. New examinations for the adult-gerontology acute
care NP, the adult-gerontology primary care NP, the adult-gerontology CNS, and the
psych/MH NP are being developed. Individual certifying bodies have established time-
lines for the implementation of these new examinations; however, the projected date for
implementation of these new certification examinations is 2012/2013. Decisions
regarding the retirement of the current examinations are also being made by the respective certification bodies. Therefore, currently certified APRNs, particularly all adult NPs
and CNSs, gerontology NPs and CNSs, and psych/MH NPs and CNSs, are urged to
remain vigilant for announcements from the certification bodies because the retirement

of these examinations will have significant impact on the options for recertification for these APRNs.

Licensure

Many states historically have used varying titles to recognize advanced practice nurses, including CRNP, ARNP, APN, and APRN. Also, many states recognized advanced practice nurses in only 1 or 2 roles. Other states recognized multiple and diverse specialties, particularly for NPs. Under the Model, APRN is identified as the legal title and credential to be granted to all advanced practice registered nurses meeting the definitional criteria. Boards of nursing (or boards of nurse-midwifery or midwifery in states where these regulate nurse midwives) are to be responsible for granting a second license to APRNs in all 4 roles: CRNA, CNM, CNS, and CNP. In addition, APRNs who meet the education and certification criteria delineated in the Model are to be licensed as independent practitioners with no regulatory requirements for collaboration, direction, or supervision.

The NCSBN at the 2008 Delegate Assembly approved the APRN Model Practice Act, which provides states with a template for developing legislation consistent with the Consensus Model. To facilitate the implementation of the Model, the NCSBN has developed a tool kit for state boards, legislators, and consumers, which includes guides for APRNs and consumers, a legislative handbook, an APRN checklist for state boards, frequently asked questions, and a video, *The Consensus Model for APRN Regulation*, posted on YouTube (http://www.ncsbn.org/2276.htm.) An interactive tool featuring a series of maps also has been developed, which enables individuals, schools, and organizations to monitor overall progress toward full implementation of the Consensus Model and changes that have been made by individual states (http://www.ncsbn.org/2567.htm).

Currently Practicing APRNs

The Model defines a future for APRN regulation. The intent of this work is not to disenfranchise currently practicing APRNs. However, as transition to this new regulatory model occurs, changes may affect currently credentialed and practicing APRNs. Grandfathering is a provision in a new law exempting those already in or part of the existing system that is being regulated. Therefore, when states adopt new eligibility requirements, practicing APRNs will be permitted to continue practicing within the state(s) of their current license. However, grandfathering cannot be mandated when an APRN moves to another state. The Model and the NCSBN APRN Model Practice Act state, however, that an APRN should be eligible for licensure in that new state if he or she is currently practicing in the role and population-focus area, is nationally certified in that role and population, and meets the education requirements of the state in which the APRN is applying that were in effect at the time the APRN completed his or her education program. Even with this recommendation, the requirement for current, national certification in the role and population is the factor that may have a significant impact on many currently practicing APRNs who are not nationally certified and who move to another state.

As mentioned previously, another change that will affect a large number of currently practicing APRNs is the implementation of new certification examinations. Recertification, particularly for adult NPs and CNSs, gerontology NPs and CNSs, and psychiatric/MH NPs and CNSs, will only be available by meeting the practice and continuing education requirements and not through retesting once the current certification examinations are retired.

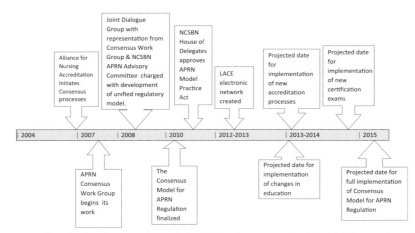

Fig. 3. Timeline for implementation of the APRN Consensus Model. AACN, American Association of Colleges of Nursing; CNM, certified nurse-midwife; CNS, clinical nurse specialist; CRNA, certified registered nurse anesthetist; DNP, Doctor of Nursing Practice; NP, nurse practitioner.

SUMMARY

The year 2015 is identified in the Model as the target date for full implementation. The organizations tasked with the implementation of the Consensus Model recognized early on that implementation must be sequential. Changes in the education programs must occur first, followed by accreditation and certification. State licensing requirements would be the last, and in most cases, the most difficult to enact because in most states it would require new legislation. However, all 4 LACE components initiated implementation processes as soon as the Model was finalized in 2008. Based on this understanding, a projected timeline for implementation was developed (**Fig. 3**). Implementation dates for specific components or processes have varied only slightly since 2008, and full implementation of the Consensus Model remains on target for 2015. As this work progresses, all APRNs and other stakeholders are strongly encouraged to remain in communication with their respective professional organizations and to monitor information posted on the LACE Web site (http://www.aprnlace.org).

The Consensus Model creates a synergistic interface between education, accreditation, certification, and licensure. When fully implemented the Consensus Model will allow APRNs to practice to the full scope of their education and more easily move from one state to another, increasing access to quality health care services for all populations. Uniform titling and credentialing will enhance APRN recognition by the public, policy makers, and other health professionals. Under the Model, APRN practice is not restricted by setting, but rather is patient-centered and based on patient needs. For example, the adult-gerontology acute care NP should not be limited to practice within the acute care hospital but rather provide care to acutely ill patients who are in the home, long-term care, or other health care setting. Likewise, the adult-gerontology primary care NP could provide increased continuity of care and follow patients into the acute care or long-term care facility to provide ongoing health maintenance and chronic disease management services.

The APRN community has been applauded for its ability to reach consensus on this landmark agreement. Endorsement by 48 national nursing organizations including all organizations with a stake in APRN regulation provides a powerful and unified front for APRNs to become full partners in reshaping the health care system as envisioned by the IOM. To reach this goal, implementation of the Consensus Model in total is critical and is dependent on the ongoing participation and collaboration among all LACE entities.

REFERENCES

1. He W, Sengupta M, Velkoff V, et al. Current population reports: 65+ in the United States. Washington, DC: U.S. Census Bureau, Government Printing Office; 2005.
2. Schoen C, Osborn R. The Commonwealth Fund 2010 International Health Policy Survey in eleven countries. 2010. Available at: http://www.Commonwealthfund. org/Surveys/2010. Accessed December 1, 2011.
3. MacDorman MF, Mathews TJ. Behind international rankings of infant mortality: how the United States compares with Europe. 2009. Available at: http://www. cdc.gov/nchs/data/databriefs/db23.htm. Accessed November 29, 2011.
4. Science Daily. National health care scorecard: United States scores 64 out of 100. 2011. Available at: http://www.sciencedaily.com/releates/2011/10/111018121836. htm. Accessed November 30, 2011.
5. Hauer KE, Durning SJ, Kernan WN, et al. Factors associated with medical students' career choices regarding internal medicine. JAMA 2008;300(10):1154–64.
6. Primary care professionals: recent supply trends, projections, and valuation of services. Testimony before the Senate Committee on Health, Education, Labor, and Pensions. Washington, DC: U.S. Government Accountability Office; 2008. GAO-08–472T.
7. Hollinghurst S, Horrocks S, Anderson E, et al. Comparing the cost of nurse practitioners and GPs on primary care. Br J Gen Pract 2006;56(528):530–5.
8. Lambing AY, Adams DL, Fox DH, et al. Nurse practitioners and physicians' care activities and clinical outcomes with an inpatient geriatric population. J Am Acad Nurse Pract 2004;16(8):343–52.
9. Lenz ER, Mundinger MO, Kane RL, et al. Primary care outcomes in patients treated by nurse practitioners or physicians: two-year follow-up. Med Care Res Rev 2004;61(3):332–51.
10. Mundinger MO, Kane RL, Lenz ER, et al. Primary care outcomes in patients treated by nurse practitioners and physicians. JAMA 2000;283(1):59–68.
11. Newhouse RP, Stanik-Hutt J, White KM, et al. Advanced practice nurse outcomes 1990-2008: a systematic review. Nurs Econ 2011;29(5):1–21.
12. The registered nurse population, findings from the March 2004 national sample survey of registered nurses. Washington, DC: U.S. Department of Health and Human Services, Health Resources and Services Administration; 2006.
13. The registered nurse population, findings from the 2008 National Sample Survey of Registered Nurses. Washington, DC: U.S. Department of Health and Human Services, Health Resources and Services Administration; 2010.
14. Institute of Medicine. The future of nursing leading change, advancing health. Washington, DC: The National Academies Press; 2011.
15. APRN Consensus Work Group, & National Council of State Boards of Nursing APRN Advisory Committee. (2008). Consensus model for APRN regulation: licensure, accreditation, certification & education. Available at: http://www.aacn.nche. edu/education-resources/APRNReport.pdf. Accessed November 28, 2011.
16. Styles MM, Schuman MJ, Bickford C, et al. Specialization and credentialing in nursing revisited: understanding issues, advancing the profession. Silver Spring (MD): American Nurses Association; 2008.

The Movement to Improve Care
The Institute of Medicine Quality Reports and Implications for the Advanced Practice Registered Nurse

Anita Finkelman, MSN, RN

KEYWORDS

- Quality improvement • Institute of Medicine • Competencies
- Advanced practice nursing • Health care profession education
- Advanced practice registered nurse

KEY POINTS

- Recent Institute of Medicine reports have highlighted the need to improve quality in health care and identified methods to create change.
- Interprofessional communication and collaboration as well as transparency are essential in creating a quality care environment.
- Care must be patient centered and evidence based to ensure quality.

Since the late 1990s there has been a movement in the United States to improve care. Nursing has been slow to embrace this movement, although this situation is improving. Nursing education was particularly slow in recognizing that the movement and the problem of health care quality related to nursing education, both undergraduate and graduate. To improve care requires efforts from practice and health care education perspectives. This article discusses the concern about the quality of care in the United States, the movement to improve, and some of the critical issues as they relate to advanced practice nursing.

INSTITUTE OF MEDICINE ESTABLISHES THE *QUALITY CHASM* SERIES

In 1997, President Clinton created the Advisory Commission on Consumer Protection and Quality in Healthcare, a temporary commission, to examine the status of health care delivery in the United States. The report from this commission, *Quality First*, recommended a more extensive examination of the health care system, because there were

Bouvé College of Health Sciences, School of Nursing, Northeastern University, 100 Robinson Hall, 360 Huntington Avenue, Boston, MA 02116, USA
E-mail address: anitawfinkelman@yahoo.com

Nurs Clin N Am 47 (2012) 251–260
doi:10.1016/j.cnur.2012.02.006
0029-6465/12/$ – see front matter © 2012 Elsevier Inc. All rights reserved.

serious problems.[1] The Institute of Medicine (IOM) was asked to take on this task. This initiative established the IOM *Quality Chasm* series of reports, which have been critical in expanding understanding of the quality of care in the US health care system.

The IOM is a nonprofit organization located in Washington, DC that was established in 1970 to provide advice to government, policy makers, health care professionals and other types of professionals, educators, and the public. The IOM cannot make laws or regulation; it can only make recommendations. Even although the IOM has the term medicine in its title, its focus is not only on medicine. The IOM reports are available free in electronic form on its Web site (http://www.iom.edu).

There is no doubt that the IOM influences policy, legislation, and funding, and affects research and practice. An example of how the IOM has affected policy and nursing is the IOM 1983 report, *Nursing Education: Public Policy and Private Actions*. This report recommended that nursing should be represented at the National Institutes of Health in order for nursing to have more influence on health care research. As a result of this recommendation, the National Institute of Nursing Research was created, although it was first established as a center as a part of the National Institutes of Health.

The IOM reports have affected recent critical nursing initiatives and publications. The American Association of Colleges of Nursing *Essentials of Baccalaureate Education for Professional Nursing Practice* highlighted the 5 IOM health care professions core competencies in the first paragraphs of its current edition and emphasizes in its recommendations the need for nurses to be involved in quality improvement (QI).[2] IOM core competencies are commented on in the *Essentials of Master's Education in Nursing*.[3] The landmark study of nursing education was also influenced by the IOM reports.[4]

THE IOM *QUALITY CHASM* REPORTS

The IOM reports on quality in health care were developed to examine the health care delivery system. The IOM uses panels of experts who are involved in a specific call to address a problem. After the work is completed, the panel is disbanded. Nurses also serve on the panels. The reports build on one another and one can see a process of development of ideas and strategies from 1 report to the next, each report trying to better examine the issues and arrive at recommendations.[5] Each report makes recommendations, which are then used by policy makers, professionals, educators, and others to guide decisions. There is greater emphasis on health care professions understanding the content of the reports and the recommendations and application to practice such as for advanced practice registered nurses (APRNs). This discussion focuses on the quality reports, but the IOM has many other reports on specific health

---

Box 1
Key IOM *Quality Chasm* reports

To Err Is Human (1999)

Crossing the Quality Chasm (2001)

Priority Areas for National Action (2003)

Disparity Reports (2003)

Public Health Reports (2004)

Keeping Patients Safe (2004)

Health Professions Education (2003)

topics such as women's health, pediatrics, emergency care, and gerontology. The key *Quality Chasm* reports are listed in **Box 1**.

To Err Is Human (1999)

This report was significant because it clearly indicated that the US health care system was not yielding the outcomes needed. It estimated that 44,000 to nearly 100,000 patients died annually in US hospitals because of errors.[6] This estimate was believed to be low at the time the data were analyzed, because hospitals did not have effective reporting and tracking systems, and there was inconsistency in terminology, for example what 1 hospital called an error might not be the same in another hospital. When the media became aware of this report, its results were highlighted on the radio and TV and in print, and the public learned about this information. This situation led to greater patient awareness of the risk of errors. Improvement has been slow.

To Err Is Human, as the first report in the series, began the process of defining critical terms such as error and safety.[6] The report describes safety as freedom from accidental injury, and error as failure of a planned action to be completed as intended or the use of a wrong plan to achieve an aim. However, there continues to be a lack of consensus on these definitions, particularly when it comes to identifying specific examples. ANPs who practice in a variety of settings and roles should use these definitions in data collection and analysis of errors.

The report also identified a critical concern: the blame game. There is too much emphasis on blame (finding the individual or individuals who made the error), when most errors are system-based. Understanding the impact of the system on errors is critical for developing effective solutions. The blame game approach has been detrimental and has limited efforts to resolve the problems. The Agency for Healthcare Research and Quality's (AHRQ) patient safety primer emphasizes that creating a safety culture is the goal, and this culture is different from the blame culture.[7] This culture is also referred to as a Just Culture. Health care organizations are trying to change their culture to meet the following safety culture criteria identified by AHRQ[7]:

- Acknowledgment of the high-risk nature of an organization's activities and the determination to achieve consistently safe operations
- A blame-free environment in which individuals are able to report errors or near misses without fear of reprimand or punishment
- Encouragement of collaboration across ranks and disciplines to seek solutions to patient safety problems
- Organizational commitment of resources to address safety concerns.

This approach does not deny that there are circumstances in which individuals play a major role in errors. When this situation occurs, after a system review, then the individual factors need to be addressed. For example, if an ANP who should know a procedure does not follow the procedure, this cannot be ignored. However, to focus only on individual blame, which has been the accepted approach for many years, is no longer acceptable.

Crossing the Quality Chasm (2001)

To Err Is Human indicated that health care providers and policy makers needed to know more about the health care delivery system and quality, and thus another examination by the IOM was begun, which resulted in the report *Crossing the Quality Chasm*.[8] This report concluded that the health care system was in need of repair and fundamental change. It was dysfunctional. Good quality was described as "providing patients with appropriate services in a technically competent manner, with good communication, shared decision-making, and cultural sensitivity."[8(p232)] This description applies to all health care providers, including ANPs. To describe a vision of quality care, the IOM identified what it called Simple Rules, describing the current approach or old rules to health care and the new approach or new rules.[8(p67)] How do these rules apply to advanced practice nursing?

- Care is based on continuous healing relationships

ANPs need to base their practice on a continuum of care and building relationships with patients and with patients' families when appropriate and when patients give their permission

- Care is customized according to patient needs and values

ANPs need to provide individualized care even when using protocols and clinical guidelines, applying evidence-based practice

- The patient is the source of control

ANPs must recognize that care is patient-centered: the patient makes all decisions about their care. The ANP may recommend, but the patient decides

- Knowledge is shared and information flows freely

ANPs work on interprofessional teams and share information through documentation and dialogue about patient care. Information is shared with the patient

- Decision making is evidence based

ANPs use evidence to back up decisions

- Safety is a system property

ANPs recognize the need to understand the impact of the health care system on safety and participate actively in the QI process

- Transparency is necessary

ANPs are open about information, for example related to reimbursement and financial issues, ensuring ethical decision making, and sharing information with patients

- Needs are anticipated

ANPs consider current patient needs but also are aware of potential needs and treatment choices

- Waste is continuously decreased

ANPs are aware of efficient use of resources (eg, financial, supplies, and other resources)

- Cooperation among clinicians is a priority.

Interprofessional teamwork is critical to ANP practice.
A typical response to this vision is "We do all of this." The conclusion from IOM is that the system does not follow these rules, and because health care providers are key elements in the system, the assumption must be made that providers are not

considering all these elements. ANPs need to integrate these elements into their daily practice, as do all health care staff.

The conclusion from the report is the identification of common care problems. When one looks at the list, it is easy to see that these are care problems that health care providers typically consider to be basic to an effective health care system. Probably, many providers assume that these are not problems in the current system, and yet the report says these are critical concerns that are not met routinely.[8]

- Failure to monitor, observe, or act
- Delay in diagnosis
- Incorrect assessment of risk
- Loss of information during transfer to other health care staff
- Failure to note faulty equipment
- Failure to carry out preoperative checks
- Deviation from an agreed protocol without clinical justification
- Failure to seek help when necessary
- Use of incorrect protocol
- Treatment given to wrong body site
- Wrong treatment plan.

With the publication of the first 2 reports, the intensive examination of the quality of the health care delivery system provides a description of the problems: development of key terminology to facilitate consistent communication; description of a vision of an improved health care system (the Rules); and identification of common care problems. The next step was to identify key goals or aims to improve health care. The aims are[8]:

1. Safe: avoiding injuries to patients from the care that is intended to help them
2. Effective: providing services based on scientific knowledge to all who could benefit and refrain from providing services not likely to benefit the patient
3. Patient-centered: providing care that is respectful of and responsive to individual patient preferences, needs, and values, ensuring that patient values guide all clinical decisions
4. Timely: reducing waits and sometimes harmful delays for both patients who receive and those who give care
5. Efficient: avoiding waste of equipment, supplies, ideas, and energy
6. Equitable: providing care that does not vary in quality because of personal characteristics such as gender, ethnicity, geographic location, and socioeconomic status.

Each one of these aims or goals relates to ANP practice and should be integral in care for all patients, regardless of the type of health care setting.

Envisioning National Healthcare Quality Report (2001)

The next step the IOM took was to use the conclusions and approaches described in earlier reports to develop a framework for health care quality.[9] The framework is a matrix that has 2 dimensions. One dimension focuses on the consumer perspective (staying healthy, getting better, living with illness or disability, and coping with the end of life), aspects that nurses have considered important in their practice. The second focuses on the health care system (safety, effectiveness, patient-centeredness, timeliness). The IOM developed a list of focus areas for monitoring care.[10] This list changes as care improves or new problems are identified. The United States now uses the matrix in the annual comprehensive national overview of quality in health care. The national monitoring of the status of quality of care is performed by the AHRQ, and the annual report is available online at the agency's Web site (http://www.ahrq.gov/qual/qrdr10.htm).

Disparity Reports

As the IOM examined health care quality, an issue arose that was difficult to accept: was there a problem with disparities in health care? This issue led to a more focused examination. The IOM completed 3 reports: *Unequal Treatment*,[11] *Guidance for the National Healthcare Disparities Report*,[12] and *Health Literacy*.[13] The first report identified that there were major problems with bias, prejudice, and stereotyping in the health care system. "Racial and ethnic minorities tend to receive a lower quality of health care than non-minorities, even when access-related factors, such as patient insurance status & income, are controlled."[11(p1)] This was a disturbing result for health care professionals, who think of themselves as caring individuals. The next step was to monitor health care disparities annually, which is also carried out by the AHRQ. The report is available on the AHRQ Web site with the quality report. The third disparity report focused on health literacy, a relatively unknown topic. The IOM describes health literacy as "the degree to which individuals obtain, process, and understand basic information and services needed to make appropriate decisions regarding their health."[13(p52)] This is an important issue for ANPs when they work with patients and their families. It is easy to make assumptions about understanding when there is a problem with full understanding. This situation can lead to errors and limit reaching effective patient outcomes.

Keeping Patients Safe (2004)

Keeping Patients Safe is part of the *Quality Chasm* series, and this report focused on nursing care.[14] It is highly supportive of nursing and identifies important concerns about the environment in which care is provided and the need to improve care. The report focused primarily on acute care nursing: (1) work design, (2) safety and central role of the nurse, (3) quality and role of the nurse, and (4) the nursing shortage. This report is an important resource to better understand nursing, for ANPs and all nurses.

Health Professions Education (2003)

After describing the problem and providing many recommendations to improve care, the IOM examined the critical issue of health profession education. Health care organizations can work to improve care, but if new health care profession graduates are not aware of the health care quality problems and improvement process and methods and do not have the competencies required to affect care positively, how can they improve care? If we ignore the input (new professionals entering the health care system), the system is always playing catch up, and improvement is difficult to achieve. Staff need to receive staff education on these topics and improve their practice, but students, both undergraduate and graduate, who will soon be staff, are a critical factor in improving care. This was the focus of the *Health Professions Education* report.[15]

Health Professions Education identified 5 core competencies for all health care professions. The *Essentials for Master's Education in Nursing* notes the importance of these 5 competencies: "In addition to broad public mandates for a reformed and responsive health care system, a number of groups are calling for changes in the ways all health professionals are educated to meet current and projected needs for contemporary care delivery."[3(p6)] The following discussion describes the IOM core competencies and their relevance to advanced practice nursing.[15]

Provide Patient-centered Care

Identify, respect, and care about patients' differences, values, preferences, and expressed needs; relieve pain and suffering; coordinate continuous care; listen to, clearly inform, communicate with, and educate patients; share decision-making and management; and continuously advocate disease prevention, wellness, and promotion of healthy lifestyles, including population health.

ANPs are involved in all aspects that influence patient-centered care and need to recognize that improved care requires that self-assessment is used to routinely determine if one is meeting these requirements to ensure patient-centered care, not only in ANP graduate programs but also after graduation in practice.

Work in Interdisciplinary/Interprofessional Teams

Cooperate, collaborate, communicate, and integrate care in teams to ensure that care is continuous and reliable.

This competency is the most difficult to accomplish. Health care profession education occurs in silos: most, if not all, nursing education is separated from other health care profession education. It takes creativity and risk to try to increase interprofessional education, but this is the only way there will be major improvement in developing effective interprofessional teams so that there is interprofessional collaborative practice.[16,17] ANPs need to work with many types of health care professions. The divide with physicians does not lead to effective teamwork and collaborative practice.

Use Evidence-based Practice

Integrate best research with clinical expertise and patient values for optimum care, and participate in learning and research activities to the extent feasible.

ANP students certainly have experience with evidence-based practice in their programs, although there is a tendency to focus on only 1 type of evidence: research. However, there are other important types of evidence: the patient's values and preferences, patient assessment (history and physical examination), and the expertise of the clinician. There also needs to be greater recognition of the need for evidence-based management (a critical area). ANPs in practice need to use best-practice evidence in their clinical decision making and in their leadership in the practice settings. It is not easy to keep current with evidence-based practice literature, but it is critical for effective patient outcomes and improved care.

Apply QI

Identify errors and hazards in care; understand and implement basic safety design principles; continually understand and measure quality of care in terms of structure, process and outcomes in relation to patient and community needs; and design and test interventions to change processes and systems of care, with the objective of improving quality.

The IOM notes that nurses should play a critical role in QI, but often nurses are not prepared to do so. Current nursing programs focus little on QI and the role of the nurse in the process. ANPs can play a critical role by first ensuring that they provide quality care and consider safety issues to prevent errors in their practice. They also need to serve as leaders to ensure that other staff keep quality care in focus, particularly nursing staff.

Use Informatics

Communicate, manage knowledge, mitigate error, and support decision-making using information technology.

Informatics is clearly part of daily practice, particularly documentation when an electronic system is used. ANPs need to be prepared to use informatics and also prepared as health care informatics changes. What are the issues around ethics and legal issues and informatics? What makes an effective documentation system? How are errors made and prevented in the emergency medicine room? What does clinical decision-making support mean? How is informatics used in QI?

THE FUTURE OF NURSING. LEADING CHANGE, ADVANCING HEALTH (2010)

This IOM report expanded on previous IOM reports on nursing and education and was also strongly influenced by the *Quality Chasm* series of reports.[18] It has also been a hot topic because of its recommendations. The report offers many important recommendations, as noted in the listing outlined later; however, the recommendation that has been discussed most is the recommendation about ANPs. It is important that all of the recommendations receive sufficient consideration and affect practice. Most nurses are not ANPs. Most nurses work daily in difficult situations to provide care. As a profession, all aspects of services need to be improved. The report is about the nursing profession and the leadership roles the profession can and should take in the health care environment, with a strong emphasis on leadership from its title to its content. The report recommendations are[18]:

1. Remove the scope-of-practice barriers
2. Expand opportunities for nurses to lead and diffuse collaborative improvement efforts
3. Implement nurse residency programs
4. Increase the proportion of nurses with baccalaureate degree to 80% by 2020
5. Double the number of nurses with a doctorate by 2020
6. Ensure that nurses engage in lifelong learning
7. Prepare and enable nurses to lead change to advance health
8. Build an infrastructure for the collection and analysis of interprofessional health care workforce data.

The IOM reports have affected how care is delivered in the United States. There is clearly need for more improvement. Some examples that have affected care and also relate to advanced practice nursing are:

- Joint Commission Annual Designation of Safety Goals

Any ANP that works in a Joint Commission accredited organization must be aware of the annual goals and follow them.

- Establishment of the Centers for Medicare and Medicaid Never Events.

This is a list of complications that may occur in a hospital setting that the Centers for Medicare and Medicaid Services (CMS) no longer cover because they are considered preventable, for example patient falls and decubiti. One can argue that they may not all be preventable, but CMS do not cover the care costs. ANPs who work in settings and have patients for whom this would apply need to be aware of these issues and also assist staff to improve care so that these complications are prevented.

- Handoffs increase errors so efforts are made to decrease handoffs (the number of times a patient changes providers or setting) and improve the process when handoffs have to be used.

ANPs are involved in handoffs. They need to consider these red flag events that require extra attention to communication and detail.

- Workarounds, times when a staff member takes a short cut to get something done, increase errors

ANPs need to avoid workarounds in their practice.

- Greater attention to QI monitoring

ANPs could take a lead role in the QI process, educating others about QI, and also better ensure that their own practice is as error free as possible, with a focus on effective patient outcomes.

- Participate in monitoring and analyzing the quality of care

ANPs can serve on QI committees and root-cause analysis teams, serve in QI roles, and assist with staff education about quality.

- Use current methods to improve practice.

ANPs should use effective patient surveillance, recognize high risk of handoffs, apply the PDSA (plan-do-study-act) cycle to resolve problems; use failure modes effects analysis to analyze safety issues; actively apply medication reconciliation to their patients; use checklists to prevent errors.

SUMMARY

"Clearly there is momentum in health care organizations (HCOs) and in government to improve health care in the United States. It is not enough to reform just health care systems; we need safety and quality strategies to resolve problems in clinical settings and strategies for government and local communities."[5(p40)] To be effective in meeting the recommendations of the *Quality Chasm* series of reports requires an understanding of the problem, best approaches to resolving the problem, commitment to improving care, collection of data, and monitoring and analyzing data to improve care. ANPs have 2 levels of responsibility: the first is with their own individual practice, to ensure quality care for their patients; second, they need to provider leadership when required in the various settings in which ANPs work to ensure quality care.

REFERENCES

1. The President's Advisory Commission on Consumer Protection and Quality in the Healthcare Industry. Quality first: better health care for all Americans. Washington, DC: US Government Printing Office; 1999.
2. The essentials of baccalaureate education for professional nursing practice. Education in Nursing. Washington, DC: American Association of Colleges of Nursing; 2008.
3. The essentials of master's education in nursing. Washington, DC: American Association of Colleges of Nursing; 2011.
4. Benner P, Sutphen M, Leonard V, et al. Educating nurses. A call for radical transformation. San Francisco (CA): Jossey-Bass; 2010.

5. Finkelman A, Kenner C. Teaching IOM: implications of the Institute of Medicine reports for nursing education. 2nd edition. Silver Spring (MD): American Nurses Association; 2009.
6. Institute of Medicine. To err is human. Washington, DC: National Academies Press; 1999.
7. Agency for Healthcare Research and Quality. Patient safety primer. 2011. Available at: http://psnet.ahrq.gov/primer.aspx?primerID=5. Accessed September 6, 2011.
8. Institute of Medicine. Crossing the quality chasm. Washington, DC: National Academies Press; 2001.
9. Institute of Medicine. Envisioning the national healthcare quality report. Washington, DC: National Academies Press; 2001.
10. Institute of Medicine. Priority areas for national action: transforming health care quality. Washington, DC: National Academies Press; 2003.
11. Institute of Medicine. Unequal treatment: confronting racial and ethnic disparities in healthcare. Washington, DC: National Academies Press; 2003.
12. Institute of Medicine. Guidance for the national healthcare disparities report. Washington, DC: National Academies Press; 2002.
13. Institute of Medicine. Health literacy: a prescription to end confusion. Washington, DC: National Academies Press; 2004.
14. Institute of Medicine. Keeping patients safe. Transforming the work environment of nurses. Washington, DC: National Academies Press; 2004.
15. Institute of Medicine. Health professions education. Washington, DC: National Academies Press; 2003.
16. Institute of Medicine. The future of nursing. Leading change, advancing health. Washington, DC: National Academies Press; 2010.
17. Interprofessional Education Collaborative Expert Panel. Core competencies for interprofessional collaborative practice: report of an expert panel. Washington, DC: Interprofessional Education Collaborative; 2011.
18. World Health Organization. Framework for action on interpersonal education & collaborative practice. Geneva (Switzerland): Author; 2010. Available at: http://www.who.int/hrh/nursing_midwifery/en/. Accessed September 6, 2011.

The Role of the Nurse Executive in Fostering and Empowering the Advanced Practice Registered Nurse

Tukea L. Talbert, DNP, RN*

KEYWORDS

- Nurse executives • Advanced nursing practice • Scope of practice
- Advanced nurse registered practice outcomes • Advanced practice registered nurse

KEY POINTS

- Nurse executives are in a unique position within the health care system to affect the use of Advanced Practice Registered Nurse and ensure that they are successfully integrated into the practice setting.
- A plan must be in place to evaluate the role that includes measurable measures of success (eg, length of stay, cost control or reduction, patient satisfaction, health care outcomes, and core measure compliance).
- Nurse executives must ensure that the role's effectiveness is supported through the development of strategies to improve and cultivate the relationship between practitioners.

Over the last several decades, the nursing profession has found itself at critical junctures to affect change in health care and make a difference in the patient experience. Once again, the nursing profession is at the proverbial "tipping point." The profession represents the largest component of the nation's health care workforce—weighing in with more than 3 million members.[1] Nurses can play a significant role in facilitating the objectives set forth in the 2010 Affordable Care Act, which is the most expansive health care overhaul since the 1965 development of the Medicare and Medicaid programs.[1] Hader[2] writes about the role of leaders and how leadership can make the best decisions to "forge forward" by being well informed regarding necessary changes to both practice and academic settings. The focus of this article is on the role of the Advanced Practice Registered Nurse (APRN) and on how nurse executives can maximize the effectiveness of the individuals in these roles. The four key areas are the executive's knowledge and self preparation, visionary leadership and

Department of Administration, 1107 West Lexington Avenue, Winchester, KY 40391, USA
* 2105 Heath Land Place, Lexington, KY 40516.
E-mail address: tl.talbert1161@yahoo.com

Nurs Clin N Am 47 (2012) 261–267
doi:10.1016/j.cnur.2012.02.007
0029-6465/12/$ – see front matter © 2012 Elsevier Inc. All rights reserved.
nursing.theclinics.com

credentialing of APRNs, strategies to reduce disconnection in health care settings between APRNs and work setting, and marketing and education about the role of the APRN.

LEADERSHIP PREPARATION: KNOWLEDGE AND POLITICAL ENGAGEMENT

In 2008, the Institute of Medicine (IOM) and the Robert Wood Johnson Foundation (RWJF) initiated work on a collaborative effort to review the state of nursing and to make recommendations to ensure that nursing is well equipped to meet the future challenges in all milieus in which the practice occurs.[1] As a result of this work, which was published in the fall of 2010, four recommendations were developed. They include (1) nurses should practice at the full extent of their training and education, (2) nurses should achieve higher levels of training and education through an enhanced education system, (3) nurses should be full and equal partners with physicians and other health care professionals with the redesign of health care, and (4) effective policy making and workforce planning necessitates an improved data collection and a better information infrastructure.[1]

One of the overarching themes from this collaborative effort was that regardless of the various practice settings, care should always be delivered in a way that is patient-centered and encompasses a culture of dignity, safety, respect, effectiveness, and efficiency. That being said, as a nurse executive, it is paramount to know what political initiatives and/or changes are on the horizon to affect nursing practice within one's own setting and outside the boundaries of one's physical health care infrastructure. More specifically, with APRN practice, the work of the IOM and RWJF has major implications for the scope of practice. The IOM committee shows that APRN practice following graduation varies extensively across the United States for reasons based on political decisions of the state and not because of their training, education, or ability.[3] In order to meet the challenges set forth in the 2010 Affordable Care Act, especially in terms of accessibility for all consumers, it is critical that APRNs not be limited in their scope of practice due to "over regulation" imposed by politicians at the state level. This issue is clearly not an issue of skill and preparation and it greatly limits the ability of APRNs to practice in a manner that will maximize the efficiency and overall effectiveness of health care systems. Nurse executives and other members of the C-suite (term referring to other chief officers, ie, CEO, CFO, & COO) must position themselves to be present, educated, and fully equipped to vote and have a voice on committees, political forums, and other steering councils that will direct the future use of APRNs and the delivery of care. Issues regarding APRN practice limitations are not only related to varying state regulations but also to reimbursement constraints for what they are educated and trained to perform.

Executives need to be aware of key driving factors that necessitate the need to rethink and redesign APRN practice. Some key reasons for change include (1) a paradigm shift from specialty to primary care, (2) a shift from acute care to community (home medicine) models of care delivery, and (3) new demands to provide more affordable care to a broader base of consumers that has resulted in an increased focus on health promotion and disease prevention. It is critical for nurse executives to know that some states have initiated steps to create compact states for licensure of APRNs. Iowa, Utah, and Texas have passed legislation that permits joining the APRN compact; however, there is no official start date for this change to occur.[4] Although, this effort is not currently executed, it represents an innovative and practical strategy to standardize the practice of the APRN across geographic boundaries, which is critical to creating a standardized model of APRN regulation and reimbursement for services.

VISIONARY LEADERSHIP AND CREDENTIALING

Leaders must create a clear vision about the role boundaries and expectations of the APRN to other members of the C-suite, board members, physicians, APRNs, and the credentialing team. This must be established when the APRN is being recruited to join an organization. Although innovation about the role is critical, scope of practice is the key driver to what can be accomplished and how the APRN is credentialed. All stakeholders need to understand key elements that dictate the practice of the APRN, including the state nurse practice act, which defines the professional scope of practice, and the individual scope of practice dictated by a specialty area (held by most APRNs).[5]

Nurse executives need to be supportive of the APRN role by educating stakeholders on the various specialties and qualifications of the APRN. Beyond holding a registered nurse license, APRNs have advanced education and clinical skills obtained through national certification and licensure that equips them to manage patient care on a broad spectrum ranging from primary and specialty care across multiple settings that include long-term care, ambulatory, and acute.

The success of the APRN and the organization will be based on alignment among the leadership expectations, scope of practice, appropriate credentialing, communication of the role boundaries or expectations, and the achievement of positive patient outcomes. If done properly at the onset of recruitment, this alignment is easily achievable. Mutually important is the on-going communication plan among all stakeholders, including bedside staff experts (ie, staff nurses) and contingent on the health care milieu, regarding role expectations and functions of the APRN in the delivery-of-care model.

STRATEGIES TO REDUCE DISCONNECTION WITHIN HEALTH CARE SETTINGS

Nurse executives must take the initiative to have pre-established steps in place to avoid the pitfalls of disconnectedness between the APRN and the organization. Frequently it is easy to forget about the key role that the APRN plays in the care delivery system regardless of the setting in which they practice. It is sometimes perceived that it is easier to discuss matters of concern, patient flow, and/or care with the physicians with whom many APRNs have their collaborative agreements. Because these individuals are typically very independent and/or practice alongside physicians, they run the risk of being overlooked or considered doing satisfactory without any added support. Some key strategies to have in place are (1) education, (2) mentorship, (3) orientation, and (4) prevention of professional isolation.

Nurse executives should ensure that the organization has educational agreements with academic health care settings and universities that are in close proximity. This is most critical for APRNs who practice in community settings and rural health care. The propensity for practitioners in these settings to experience isolation and lack of connectivity is greater due to limited resources. Through educational agreements, individuals can be privy to educational offerings, classes for furthering their educational degrees, mentorship opportunities, and the development of a network for professional support and resources. Avoidance of isolation in rural settings is identified as a key strategy to retain practitioners in those settings.[6]

In conjunction with the educational opportunities, nurse executives need to develop partnerships with academic health care settings to provide clinical exposure and experience for APRNs. This will provide additional opportunities for further development of clinical skills as well as serve as another professional network for individuals that can facilitate on-going mentoring.

Orientation is another major source of satisfaction and connectivity. It is critical that individuals are oriented to the organization in a formal process that includes reporting hierarchy and organizational chart, role boundaries and expectations (credentialing privileges), resources, evaluation process, policy and procedures, and their individual preceptorship. It is paramount for nurse executives to work with key stake holders in the organization to ensure that the orientation is in place before the start of employment. With the recruitment process, it is essential to market the education, mentorship, and orientation to potential team members. Most of the time, APRNs are chosen based solely on what they have to offer and what the institution can offer in regards to their clinical expertise and/or experience. The nurse executive must raise the bar among the entire team and offer a more comprehensive package for potential new APRN team members. The ulterior objectives are to recruit and retain the best candidates for the position.

Nurse executives must take the appropriate steps to prevent APRNs from experiencing professional isolation. This is particularly an issue in rural health care settings and smaller community health care venues in nonurban locations. Individuals often feel that they have inadequate resources for referrals, resources, and professional advice. Several strategies could be implemented and they are highly contingent on the practice setting. One, there should be a reputable, dependable electronic health record that is well supported by an information technology infrastructure. Ideally, the electronic health record allows the practitioner to share records as needed with others in the organization to provide a continuum of care for patients. Two, pharmaceutical support for drug interactions, calculations, and substitutions is a vital component of daily practice. Again, this is something that generally goes unnoticed by organizations especially if the practitioner practices outside the boundaries of the hospital itself. Three, practitioners need to have the ability to refer patients to specialists especially for the more problem-prone areas such as pain management for chronic pain issues, psychiatric patient conditions, oncology services, and surgical subspecialties. The need for these services is contingent on the health care milieu that the APRN practices. Four, the most basic strategy, but commonly overlooked, is giving the practitioner a voice by ensuring that they are brought to the table to discuss critical issues that impact patient care, policy development, and changes to care delivery. Frequently, APRNs are not represented on key hospital committees. In lieu of the APRN, the physicians that they share collaborative agreements with often represent the team and/or the area in which they practice. This often sends a strong message of exclusion and individuals find themselves on the outside looking in and/or simply disconnected and disinterested. It is critical that the nurse executive ensure that these individuals are present during times of critical discussions that result in major decisions. When these decisions are made in tandem with the practitioner, it sends a message about the level of importance of these individuals along with the value they bring to the delivery of care.

Many of these suggestions are supported in the literature as strategies to keep APRNs connected to organizations especially if they work in rural health care settings. Conger and Plager[6] investigated the reasons why APRNs who work specifically in rural health care settings experience disconnectedness with their work settings. This topic was and continues to be vital when looking at the scarcity of providers and its impact on access to health care especially in rural nonurban settings. The 2010 Affordable Care Act will only make it more necessary for nurse executives and other members of the C-suite to be more cognizant of supply and demand challenges across all health care continuums within their organization and enterprise-wide. Access will continue to be a hot topic and the hospital leadership will be charged with the task of looking at fiscally sound strategies to meet the demands of an aging population that is shifting care outside the traditional boundaries of acute care settings. Nurse executives must take the initiative and operate ahead of the curve to meet the challenges of a dynamic health care environment that has yet to culminate in one of its most monumental overhauls in history.

EDUCATION AND MARKETING

To maximize the marketing and use of the APRN role, one must have a good understanding of what the APRN is capable of performing. At this juncture, it is critical to highlight that the role was widely pioneered and developed in the United States to address issues such as access to care, health care cost, shortages among primary care physicians, and changing health care needs.[7,8] These reasons for the development of the role still exist today at a more critical level.

Today, it is critical for the nurse executive to communicate the depth of the scope of practice of the APRN. Often times, this is not known to many within and outside the health care milieu. In summary, the APRN can do the following: assess health status, diagnose, develop and implement a treatment plan, and conduct a follow-up evaluation of patient status.[5]

When marketing the role of the APRN, it is significant to share the cost-effectiveness of the role. The median compensation for primary care physicians and internal medicine providers ranges from $198,000 to $205,000, respectively.[9] The average early 2011 salary for nurse practitioners (NPs) across all specialties practicing full-time is $91,310, with the average full-time total income of $98,760.[10] Nurse practitioner preparation currently costs 20% to 25% of the cost of physician preparation.[10] TennCare, Tennessee's state managed care organization, stated that NPs delivered health care at 23% below the average cost of other primary care providers with a 21% reduction in hospital inpatient rates and 24% reduced lab use rates compared with physicians.[11] Chen and colleagues[12] showed that NP-managed care was associated with reduced overall drug costs for inpatients. A broader study conducted in a large health maintenance organization setting showed that adding an NP to the practice drastically increased the number of patients seen by the physician. The NP doubled the number of patients being seen and increased revenue by $1.28 per member per month, which was equivalent to approximately $1.65 million per 100,000 enrollees per year.[13]

Although the literature regarding the cost-effectiveness of using APRNs is positive, it is not the only advantage that they bring to the table. The most valuable aspect of the APRN is not solely based on productivity from a cost perspective but more so the impact they make at the point of care. For more than three decades, evidence has shown the clinical significance and impact of their care. Spitzer and colleagues[14] conducted a randomized controlled trial that showed comparable mortality rates, patient satisfaction, and health care outcomes between patients managed by NP and physician care groups. Quality of care was similar and patient satisfaction was high in both groups. Horrocks and colleagues[15] conducted a meta-analysis of findings from randomized trials that indicated that patients who received NP managed care were more satisfied and had better quality of care in comparison to those who received physician care. These study findings also showed no difference in health care outcomes between the two groups of patients. Ohman-Strickland and colleagues[16] conducted a study of 46 practices and measured compliance to the American Diabetes Association (ADA) guidelines. They found that practices with NPs were more likely to perform better on quality measures and meet targets for lipid levels. More specifically, NPs who practice in the emergency department (ED) can directly impact length of stay and turn-around time, freeing up physicians to see more critically ill patients.[17] A major subsequent benefit of reducing total turn-around time is reduction of the overall risk to the facility that results from patients leaving the ED and not receiving medical screens due to lengthy wait times.

In summary, the APRN role has many marketable benefits. These practitioners not only save money from a salary and education perspective, they directly affect revenue for health care systems. Most important, the care provided by APRNs is comparable to that of a physician provider and health care outcomes are just as good if not better in some instances. As a nurse executive, the APRN role would be an easy sale. The evidence supports the advantages of the role and executives would be remiss to not ensure that all attributes of the role are fully disclosed to key stakeholders up to and including the board of trustees and physicians who may be potential partners with practitioners.

SUMMARY

Nurse executives are truly in a unique position within the health care system to affect the use of APRNs and ensure that they are successfully integrated into the practice setting. Health care organizations are in place to serve communities and to ensure the health of communities. Nurse executives know that the essence of professional nursing practice is the nurse-patient relationship. This relationship is the cornerstone of the success of the healing aspect of the consumer-provider interaction. Although the training, education, and subsequent practice of the APRN is very advanced and complex, the crux of the effectiveness of what the nurse does is based on the fundamentals of nursing practice taught in every undergraduate course.

Nurse executives must take the initiative to ensure that APRNs are fully integrated into the health care organization. They must ensure that all stakeholders understand the role and the expected outcomes. Success of the individual will be contingent on senior leadership supporting individuals in the role by giving them a voice and by educating others on the APRN role and positive health care outcomes associated with the role. Clarity must be established by the nurse executive from the point of recruitment, orientation, and the hiring of the APRN. An evaluation plan must be in place that includes measurable measures of success (eg, length of stay, cost control or reduction, patient satisfaction, health care outcomes, core measure compliance). Last and certainly not least, nurse executives must ensure that the APRN role's effectiveness is supported through the development of strategies to improve and cultivate the relationship between practitioners. In closing, Conway-Welch, the nursing dean at Vanderbilt in Nashville, TN, sums up the ultimate goal for health care reform that all nurse executives need to embrace as they move forward. Conway-Welch stated, "The right provider giving the right care at the right time to the right patient for the right reasons at the right cost in the right setting, for the right reimbursement."[18] Although this sounds like a logical and easy strategy to execute, it is no small task. Nurse executives must equip themselves to ensure that APRNs are brought to the table to help ensure that the objectives of the 2010 Affordable Care Act can be met: all patients have access to care and all providers are included in the payment infrastructure for the care that they provide.

REFERENCES

1. IOM. The future of nursing: leading change, advancing health. Washington, DC: The National Academy Press; 2010.
2. Hader R. Forging forward. Nurs Manag 2011;42(3):34–8.

3. IOM. The future of nursing: focus on scope of practice. Washington, DC: The National Academies Press; 2011.
4. Watson E, Hillman H. Advanced practice registered nursing: licensure, education, scope of practice, and liability issues. J Leg Nurse Consult 2010;21(3):25–9.
5. Swenson DE. Advanced registered nurse practitioners: standards of care and the law. J Leg Nurse Consult 2006;17(4):3–6.
6. Conger MM, Plager KA. Connectedness versus disconnectedness. Online J Rural Nurs Health Care 2008;8(1):24–38.
7. Griffin M, Melby V. Developing an advanced nurse practitioner service in emergency care: attitudes of nurses and doctors. Blackwell Publishing Ltd; 2006.
8. Standards of practice. Washington, DC: American Academy of Nurse Practitioners; 2007. Available at: http://www.aanp.org+standards+of+Practice. Accessed October 22, 2011.
9. American Medical Group Association (2009). 2009 physician compensation survey. Available at: http://www.cehKasearch.com/compensation/amga. Accessed October 22, 2011.
10. American Academy of Nurse Practitioner (2010). Nurse practitioner cost-effectiveness. Washington, DC. Available at: http://www.aanp.org/NR/rdonlyres/34E7FF57-EO71-4014-B554-FF02B82F2/o/Qualityof. Accessed October 22, 2011.
11. Spitzer R. The Vanderbilt experience. Nurs Manag 1997;28(3):38–40.
12. Chen C, McNeese-Smith D, Cowan M, et al. Evaluation of a nurse practitioner led care management model in reducing inpatient drug utilization and costs. Nurs Econ 2009;27(3):160–8.
13. Burl J, Bonner A, Rao M. Demonstration of the cost-effectiveness of a nurse practitioner/physician team in primary care teams. HMO Pract 1994;8(4):156–7.
14. Spitzer WO, Sackett DL, Sibley JC, et al. The Burlington randomized trial of the nurse practitioner. N Engl J Med 1974;290(5):251–6.
15. Horrocks S, Anderson E, Salisbury C. Systematic review of whether nurse practitioners working in primary care can provide equivalent care to doctors. BMJ 2002;324:819–23.
16. Ohman-Strickland PA, Orzan AJ, Hudson SV, et al. Quality of diabetes in care in family medicine practices: influence of nurse practitioners and physicians assistants. Ann Fam Med 2008;6(1):14–22.
17. Canadian Nurse Practitioner Initiative (2005a). Nurse practitioners in the emergency department, CNPI, Ottawa. Available at: http://www.cnpi.ca/documents/pdf/NP_emergency-department_2005_e.pdf. Accessed December 18, 2006.
18. Carlson J. Rethinking nursing. Mod Healthc 2009;39:6–7.

The Role of the Advanced Practice Registered Nurse in Ensuring Evidence-Based Practice

Marthe J. Moseley, PhD, RN, CCNS[a,b,*]

KEYWORDS

- Advanced practice registered nurse (APRN) • Evidence-based practice (EBP)
- Advanced practice role • Nursing

KEY POINTS

- A current advanced practice registered nurse (APRN) evidence-based practice (EBP) model is the ACE (Academic Center for Evidence-Based Practice) Star Model: discovery, summary, translation, integration, and evaluation.
- EBP is a process for making an informed clinical decision.
- The 3 APRN competencies necessary to apply EBP to clinical decision making are construction of searches, use of the strongest levels of evidence, and use of valid instruments to critically appraise clinical practice guidelines.

The APRN is important in role-modeling and ensuring EBP engagement at the point of care. As early as 2002, national competencies were being formulated for use not only in institutions of higher education but also in the clinical arena. This article describes a process of formulation of national competencies for EBP, specific to the APRN level. The model that is described is the ACE Star Model. Select competencies that were delineated through the process of national consensus using the ACE Star Model are discussed for the APRN role. Personal reflection is encouraged based on an understanding of an EBP skill set. Once competencies are discussed, the formation of a personal action plan is suggested to identify personal competencies for EBP. In addition, identification of EBP competency deficits targets further work on the action plan in areas in which the APRN may lack skills.

THE ACE STAR MODEL

The first annual Summer Institute on Evidence-Based Practice, featured in 2002, focused on foundational and intermediate EBP concepts.[1] The conference participants

Disclosures: none.
[a] Office of Nursing Service, Veterans Healthcare Administration, 810 Vermont Avenue NW, Washington, DC 20420, USA
[b] Rocky Mountain University of Health Professions, 561 East 1860 South, Provo, UT 84606, USA
* 101 Bikeway Lane, San Antonio, TX 78231.
E-mail address: Marthe.Moseley@va.gov

Nurs Clin N Am 47 (2012) 269–281
doi:10.1016/j.cnur.2012.02.004   **nursing.theclinics.com**
0029-6465/12/$ – see front matter Published by Elsevier Inc.

completed surveys about their opinion of EBP competencies and the integration into various nursing roles including practice, education, research, quality improvement, and administration. The conference participants' responses were then clustered into like groups that included staff nurses, educators, APRNs, nurse researchers, and quality improvement (QI) managers/nurse administrators. At this first Summer Institute, concurrent sessions provided guidance and assistance to the participants to develop EBP nursing competencies related to the 5 points of the then recently developed ACE Star Model.[2] The model included 5 points: original research (currently described as discovery), evidence summary (currently named summary), translation, implementation (currently renamed integration), and evaluation (**Table 1**). As the model was refined, new titles were used to describe points on the model (**Fig. 1**). Eighty-two EBP competency worksheets were collected from the participants. The participant breakdown by role is shown in **Table 2**.

Following the coding of each of the noted competencies, the data analysis project team then used a consensus-forming expert panel approach to establish and verify statements of EBP competencies, leveled across all identified roles.[3,4] Initial content analysis of the 82 competencies worksheets was conducted by 2 doctorally prepared nurses and a doctoral nursing student. The team then edited the competencies for duplication and filled in the gaps in the list and formatted the list into a Likert scale (forced choice, strongly agree to strongly disagree) for later use with an expert panel.

EBP COMPETENCIES

The educational competencies were further developed at a national consensus in July of 2004 at the first Invitational EBP Roundtable held in conjunction with the 2004 Summer Institute for Evidence-Based Practice.[2] The goal of the roundtable was to define essential competencies incorporated into nursing education programs at the undergraduate, graduate, and doctoral levels, recognizing that specification of competencies could be developed for clinical nurse specialist (CNS), nurse practitioner (NP), administrators, educators, and other specialty roles.[5]

Using identified competencies from the Master's level section developed at the National Consensus Roundtable,[5] selected competencies (6 of 32) are identified for further discussion and are seen as foundational for the APRN role and vital for application of EBP in the clinical setting. These selected competencies are listed in **Table 3**.

Table 1 ACE Star Model with point labels and descriptions			
Point #	Label	Description	Current Label
1	Original research	New knowledge is discovered through primary research	Discovery
2	Evidence summary	All research is synthesized into a single, meaningful statement of the state of the knowledge	Summary
3	Translation	Research evidence is translated into clinical recommendations	Translation
4	Implementation	Individual, organizational, and environmental practices are changed through formal and informal channels	Integration
5	Evaluation	Impact of change is measured at various endpoints and outcomes	Evaluation

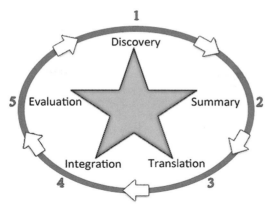

Fig. 1. ACE Star Model of knowledge transformation.

The first of the 3 selected competencies are used within the context of posing clinical questions and searching for the answers to those clinical questions.[6] The next 3 competencies are part of what makes the APRN such an important role model for the nursing team to ensure the application of EBP in the clinical setting. The first 3 competencies are discussed within the context of the process of asking and answering the clinical question.

ASKING AND ANSWERING THE CLINICAL QUESTION

Numerous sources use formats to engage in the process of asking and answering a clinical question. Strauss[7] suggests 5 steps for EBP: (1) converting the need for information into an answerable question; (2) finding the best evidence with which to answer that question; (3) critically appraising the evidence for its validity, impact, and applicability; (4) integrating the evidence with clinical expertise and the patient's values; and (5) evaluating the effectiveness and efficiency of the process. The University of Washington[8] offers 4 steps for the EBP process: (1) start with the patient, because clinical problems and questions arise out of patient care; (2) translate the clinical questions into a searchable question using PICO (population, intervention, comparison, outcome); (3) decide on the best type of study to address the question; (4) perform a literature search in the appropriate source(s). The Center for Evidence-Based Medicine, Toronto,[9] has an instructional Web site that is tutorial in nature and guides the user through the steps of formulating the clinical question.

Table 2		
Nursing role for EBP competencies		
Role	**Count**	**Subrole**
Education	15	Undergraduate Graduate PhD
Practice	30	Staff nurse APRN
Research	22	N/A
QI/Administration	15	N/A

Abbreviation: N/A, not applicable.

Table 3
Selected EBP competencies for the Master's level

Star Point		Competency
1	Discovery	Construct searches
1	Discovery	Use the strongest level of evidence
3	Translation	Use valid instruments to critically appraise clinical practice guidelines
4	Integration	Provide leadership for integrating EBP in clinical practice
4	Integration	Serve as an EBP mentor to other health care team members
5	Evaluation	Communicate results

Similar to the steps in the references mentioned earlier, the EBP "getting started" process offers a similar pathway to answering the clinical question (**Fig. 2**). Throughout the development of curriculum and the subsequent teaching in both graduate-level and doctoral-level nursing programs, the steps in this EBP process have been used as a graphic to initiate finding the answer to the question and then making the plan to incorporate EBP into practice for APRNs.

APRNs who use the EBP steps to get started provide role models for behavior that will encourage team members to use good EBP practices and thereby strengthen EBP competencies. As the APRN empowers other members of the health care team, specifically other staff nurse team members, these team members become engaged in the EBP journey and then begin to ask their own clinical questions.

Being able to ask clinical questions assumes that the clinical environment is conducive to inquiry and promotes critical thinking and clinical questioning. If this is not the case in the current clinical environment, then establishing the culture of respect and trust is a priority, with the movement toward clinical inquiry beginning at a later date.

Difficulties with staging a clinical question have been encountered by even the brightest APRNs; just promoting questioning can usually be accomplished through the use of an educator with a strong EBP background or through the use of a facilitator. Another option to promote questioning is to explore various formats for posing clinical questions. Historically, formats for posing clinical questions began with the use of the DOE (disease-oriented evidence) format. As questioning formats became more sophisticated, the format of POEMS (patient-oriented evidence that matters) became

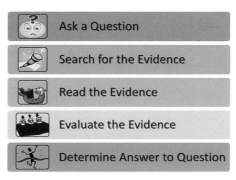

Fig. 2. Getting started: steps in the EBP process.

the favored format. Frequently used formats also include SPICE (setting, population, intervention, comparison, evaluation), ECLIPSE (expectation, client, location, intervention, professionals, service), and the ever popular PICO (and the often used PICOT [population, intervention, comparison, outcome, time] format). **Table 4** delineates each format, definitions for the format of each letter, and a sample question using the specific format.

Slawson and colleagues[10] described the classic attributes of useful information used by physicians to pose clinical questions that had relevance to everyday practice: the validity of the information and the work required to obtain it. They introduced the POEMs format, which became more popular than the DOE format of questioning. DOE deals with end points, such as changes in laboratory values or other measures of response.[11] Although the results of DOE sometimes parallel the results of POEMs, the results do not always correspond. The POEMs format deals with outcomes of importance to patients, which include changes in morbidity, mortality, or quality of life.[11]

Table 4
Clinical question formats with sample questions

Format		Definition of Format for Each Letter	Sample Question Using Specified Format
DOE	D	Disease	Sepsis diagnosis
	O	Oriented	Early identification in the ED
	E	Evidence that matters	Survival with early treatment
POEMS	P	Patient	ED patient
	O	Oriented	Early identification of sepsis
	E	Evidence that	Survival with early treatment
	Ms	Matters	Functional status at baseline 30 days after hospital discharge
SPICE	S	Setting	ED
	P	Population	Patients with sepsis
	I	Intervention	Early identified patients
	C	Comparison	Routine identification
	E	Evaluation	Functional status at baseline 30 days after hospital discharge
ECLIPSE	E	Expectation	Functional status at baseline 30 days after hospital discharge
	C	Client	Patients with sepsis
	L	Location	ED
	I	Intervention	Early screening
	P	Professionals	Registered nurses
	Se	Service	Inpatient services (ED and ICU)
PICO	P	Population	Patients in the ED
	I	Intervention	Early identification of sepsis
	C	Comparison	Routine identification
	O	Outcome	Functional status at baseline 30 days after hospital discharge
PICOT	P	Population	Patients in the ED
	I	Intervention	Identification of sepsis
	C	Comparison	Routine identification
	O	Outcome	Functional status at baseline 30 days after hospital discharge
	T	Time	Earliest time possible to identify

Abbreviations: ED, emergency department; ICU, intensive care unit.

Booth[12] devised the mnemonic SPICE, and proposed 2 noteworthy changes from the classic PICO format (discussed later). Booth[12] recognized that clinical questioning is a social science and thus chose to split the population component into setting and perspective. This splitting into component parts validates the understanding that clinical questioning is subjective and requires definition of a specific stakeholder's view that is the focus. The second change noted in the SPICE format encourages a broader evaluation framework indicated by the component outcomes, incorporating other concepts such as outputs and impact. This format of posing clinical questions is favored by librarians.

The ECLIPSE format was developed to address questions from the health policy and management area.[13] For those who use this format for posing clinical questions, it is useful because this format starts with the end in mind (E for expectation).

Probably the most familiar format for composing clinical questions is PICO.[14,15] The PICO framework is primarily centered on therapy questions, and is thought to be less suitable for representing other types of clinical information needs.[16] However, it is the most commonly taught format as well as the most commonly used format in many hospital settings.

The key to perfecting the ability to write a clinical question is to practice, practice, practice. The ability to question accomplishes different tasks. Kowalski[17] offers several benefits of questioning: stimulate the brain, create an exchange, discover knowledge or issues, encourage listening, provide the opportunity for acknowledgment, and lead the process of discovery. There are reasons for posing clinical questions in a specified format. Some of these reasons include the realization that questioning helps focus scarce learning time on evidence that is relevant to patients' clinical needs; questioning can suggest effective search strategies or suggest the forms that useful answers might take; and questioning in specific standardized formats helps to communicate more clearly with colleagues. Significant changes in practice begin with posing 1 clinical question at a time.[18]

The second step in getting started is to search for the evidence. The ability to construct searches is one of the APRN competencies listed in **Table 3**. Electronic search engines, Web sources for EBP guidelines, professional organizations, and the literature are all possible places to begin the search. The search is determined based on what the question focuses on, thus emphasizing how important it is to master the skill of posing clinical questions.

PubMed[19] is free full-text archive of biomedical and life sciences journal literature at the US National Institutes of Health's National Library of Medicine. Begin with the link to the Web site (http://www.ncbi.nlm.nih.gov/pubmed/). Keywords are determined by the constructed clinical question and are then used to search the database. The searcher is able to browse by title, volume, and issue. Other searches are accomplished by targeting an author, a specific journal, or an article. Other options of search engines are available, for example the Cumulative Index to Nursing and Allied Health Literature (CINAHL), and Proquest; however, some access for searching requires a subscription and the entry site is usually password protected. At some point near the beginning of the search, the option to limit the search is determined. Limits include the type of manuscript, publication language, species, gender, subsets, ages, and text options. The limits set on the search are determined by the searcher.

The task of searching the evidence for most APRNs is not difficult. Determining what is important to read or not to read is often confusing. Traditional methods of choosing what to read have been based on some of the following criteria: who the author is, what the journal is, what year the publication was printed, as well as personal opinion in determining the choice of materials to read.

In a study on adopting evidence-based practice in clinical decision making, Majid and colleagues[20] used the premise that evidence-based practice provided nurses with a method to use critically appraised and scientifically proven evidence for delivering quality health care to specific populations. The objective of this study was to explore nurses' awareness of, knowledge of, and attitude toward EBP and factors likely to encourage or create barriers to adoption of EBP. Information sources used by nurses and their literature searching skills were investigated through distribution of 2100 copies of the questionnaire, with a return rate of 1486 completed forms, resulting in a 70.8% response rate. Regarding self-efficacy of EBP-related abilities, the nurses perceived themselves to possess moderate levels of skills; however, for literature searching, nurses were using basic search features. The investigators concluded that, although nurses showed a positive attitude toward EBP, certain barriers were hindering their smooth adoption.

The volume of literature alone is daunting when considering what to read. In addition, not wanting the reading of the literature to become a barrier to the adoption of EBP, tips for choosing what to read as well as having an understanding of the use of evidence pyramids is important in the next step of getting started. Using the strongest level of evidence is another Master's level EBP competency noted in **Table 3**.

Once the APRN has accessed a database with inputted search terms, the search is deployed. Articles found in that search are revealed both as a number count and also as individual listings. A systematic strategy is used to narrow the search to the articles that will be read. Inclusion criteria determine which articles are kept and which are not. Various portions from the pool of captured articles are compared with the inclusion criteria. This comparison is accomplished by reviewing the title words to determine which articles will be excluded. This step is repeated by reviewing the abstracts of the articles and then reviewing the article itself. Some articles, once they are read, will still be excluded from the review. In a systematic review of APRN outcomes by Newhouse and colleagues,[21] the method of the search to determine what to read and how to narrow articles by the inclusion criteria provides a good example for an APRN learning how to choose what to include (**Table 5**).

Another consideration when determining which articles to read is that of knowing the importance of the evidence pyramids. There are numerous evidence pyramids that can provide a context for choosing which articles to read, especially if there is limited time for reading coupled with a need to answer a clinical question quickly. As the evidence pyramid is ascended, the amount of available literature decreases; however, the literature increases in its relevance to the clinical setting.[22] The evidence

Table 5
Exclusion strategy based on inclusion criteria

Step	No. of Articles Included at This Step	Following Review with Rationale (If Applicable) No. of Articles Excluded
Electronic databases (MEDLINE, CINAHL, Proquest)	27,993	Duplicates: 1734
Title review	26,259	19,146
Abstract review	7113	5425
Article review	1688	1581
Aggregated outcomes	69	Did not have aggregated outcomes: 34 CNS and NPs were combined: 4

pyramid shows a hierarchy of strength of evidence. The weaker, more prevalent evidence is at the bottom of the pyramid and the stronger, rarer, evidence is at the top. Some examples include the University of Virginia Health Sciences Library (**Fig. 3**), Medical Research Library (**Fig. 4**), and the evidence pyramid used in the substance abuse field (**Fig. 5**).

The next step in EBP is evaluating the evidence. After completing the search, critical appraisal skills are needed to evaluate the evidence. The importance of critical appraisal is to determine 3 purposes: the issues of validity, clinical importance, and applicability (**Table 6**).[23] Critical appraisal is the process of systematically examining the research evidence to determine its validity, results, and relevance before using it to inform a decision.

Each type of article has an exact match for a critical appraisal tool. Matching the article to the specific type of critical appraisal tool is important in the step of examining, and thus evaluating, the evidence. **Table 7** lists various types of articles with the matched critical appraisal tool as well as a link to the tool. This list is not all-inclusive, but serves to give numerous examples to familiarize the APRN with the process of matching the article to the appropriate tool.

It is possible that, for a specific type of article, there may not be a specific critical appraisal tool available. The APRN would recognize that a match cannot be found and thus would skip this step and move on to the next step in the EBP process. The APRN would be assured that the critical appraisal step was attempted, knowing how important this step is in the EBP process.

When the APRN initiates the process of critical appraisal, the article is read from a different perspective than for a typical read. This perspective is that of a judge. Guided by the questions from the critical appraisal tool, the APRN culls for the answer in the article and then scores the tool as prompted and as appropriate. For many APRNs, the step of critical appraisal is new and is also time consuming. The APRN develops this competency over time and with practice. This step remains important; for example, use of valid instruments to critically appraise clinical practice guidelines is one of the APRN competencies listed in **Table 3**. The process of critical appraisal for the variety of study designs possible is not the intent of this article and thus is not included.

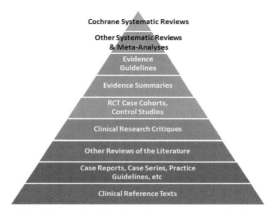

Fig. 3. Pyramid modified from "Navigating the Maze," University of Virginia, Health Sciences Library. http://healthlinks.hsl.washington.edu/ebp/images/pyramid_50_pct.gif. RCT, randomized controlled trial.

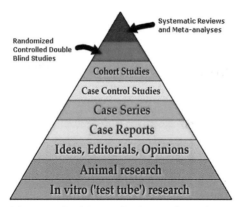

Fig. 4. Pyramid adapted from Medical Research Library of Brooklyn. http://libpweb.nus.edu.sg/mlb/g/pyramidevid2.JPG.

A systematic review[24] was undertaken of 121 published critical appraisal tools sourced from 108 papers and then classified according to the study design for which they were intended. Their items were then classified by criteria based on their intent. Commonly occurring items were identified. Eighty-seven percent of critical appraisal tools were specific to a research design; however, there was considerable variability in the items contained in the critical appraisal tools. Twelve percent of available tools were developed using specified empirical research. Forty-nine percent of the critical appraisal tools summarized the quality appraisal into a numeric summary score. Few critical appraisal tools had documented evidence of reliability of use or validity of their items. Guidelines regarding administration of the tools were provided in only 43% of the cases. There was considerable variability in intent, components, construction, and psychometric properties of those published critical appraisal tools. The conclusions were that there is no gold standard critical appraisal tool for any study design, nor is there any widely accepted generic tool that can be applied equally well across study types. Thus, interpretation of critical appraisal of research reports currently needs to be considered in light of the properties and intent of the critical appraisal tool chosen for the task.

The next step in EBP is to determine the answer to the posed question. The answer is gleaned from the best research evidence. Moving beyond the initial impression of what the answer might be, the APRN needs to account for the essence of the definition

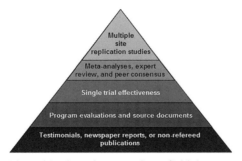

Fig. 5. Evidence pyramid used in the substance abuse field. http://www.sph.umich.edu/mi-info/10-ebph/pyramid.gif.

Table 6
Practical meaning of the purposes of critical appraisal

Purpose	Purpose Meaning
Validity	Can I trust this information?
Clinical Importance	If the information is true, will the use of this information make an important difference?
Applicability	Can I use the information in this instance or with my patient population?

of EBP. The APRN must take into context the APRN's clinical expertise and the patient's values and preferences.[25] There are numerous definitions of EBP; however, most account for 3 essential elements: best available evidence, clinician expertise, and patient values.

Three competencies have been described for the APRN: construction of searches, use of the strongest level of evidence, and use of valid instruments to critically appraise clinical practice guidelines. In addition, steps of action have been described to assist the APRN who may not have expertise in these EBP competencies. Next, this article discusses the competency to provide leadership for integrating EBP in clinical practice, serving as an EBP mentor to other health care team members, and the communication of results.

In the implementation of EBP, strategies central to the role of the CNS were studied by Muller and colleagues.[26] A hospital organization served to fully integrate the role of the CNS in the implementation of EBP. The CNS was responsible for the identification and remedy of system-wide challenges to optimal quality care, mentorship of clinical nurses both as clinicians and as leaders, and enhancement of interdisciplinary partnerships. The CNS role was integrated into the nursing department as the knowledge keepers, knowledge seekers, and knowledge disseminators. The CNS proactively developed and enhanced interdisciplinary partnerships through systematic educational sessions and the use of outcome measurement tools. The CNSs availed themselves of resources that included role development seminars, individual mentoring, and standardization of role expression across service lines. In addition, the CNSs developed and implemented outcome measurement tools to quantify CNS contributions,

Table 7
Articles by type matched to critical appraisal tool noted by hyperlink

Type (and Subtype) of Article	Abbreviation	Type of Critical Appraisal Tool	Web Link for Critical Appraisal Tool
Systematic review	SR	Critical appraisal tool for SR	http://www.cebm.net/index.aspx?o=1157
Randomized control trial	RCT	—	—
1 Therapy		Critical appraisal tool for therapy	http://www.cebm.net/index.aspx?o=1157
3 Prognosis	—	Critical appraisal tool for prognosis	http://www.cebm.net/index.aspx?o=1157
4 Diagnosis		Critical appraisal tool for diagnosis	http://www.cebm.net/index.aspx?o=1157
Clinical practice guidelines	CPG	Critical appraisal tool for CPGs	http://www.agreetrust.org

standardizing role implementation. This dedication of resources resulted in a significant number of unit-based and system-wide CNSs serving as significant support to the clinical nurse's practice and leadership development.

Another example that gives evidence to the APRN leadership, mentoring, and communication competency in promoting EBP are the influencing factors among frontline nurses from a cross-sectional survey.[27] This study identified factors influencing APRNs contribution to promoting EBP among frontline nurses. Care should be evidence based. Nurses experience challenges in implementing EBP. A survey of 855 APRNs working in 87 hospital/primary care settings in the United Kingdom were examined for their understanding of EBP, sources of evidence used, ways of working with frontline nurses, perceived impact on frontline nurses, skills in EBP, and barriers to promoting EBP. APRNs used different sources of evidence, engaged in various activities to promote EBP, and had a positive influence on frontline nurses' practice. APRNs were well placed as clinical leaders to promote EBP by frontline nurses because the APRNs were opinion leaders and influenced the practice of frontline nurses.

Gerrish and colleagues[28] studied the role of the APRN in knowledge brokering as a means of promoting EBP among clinical nurses. The aim of the study was to identify approaches used by APRNs to promote EBP among clinical nurses. Barriers were encountered at individual and organizational levels. These barriers hindered clinical nurses in their ability to deliver EBP. APRNs are well placed to promote EBP through interactions with clinical nurses. A multiple instrumental case study of 23 APRNs from hospital and primary care settings was undertaken. Data collection comprised interviews and observation of APRNs as well as interviews with clinical nurses and other health care professionals. APRNs acted as knowledge brokers in promoting EBP among clinical nurses. Knowledge management and promoting the uptake of knowledge were key components of knowledge brokering. Knowledge management was composed of different elements (**Box 1**). APRNs promoted the uptake of evidence by developing the knowledge and skills of clinical nurses through role-modeling, teaching, clinical problem solving, and facilitating change. The APRN role in knowledge brokering was complex, multifaceted, and extended beyond the knowledge management, linkage, and capacity building identified in the literature to include active processes of problem solving and facilitating change.

EBP is a process for making an informed clinical decision. Three selected competencies needed by the APRN to apply EBP to clinical decision making include construction of searches, use of the strongest levels of evidence, and use of valid instruments to critically appraise clinical practice guidelines. EBP is about using the best research evidence. When integrated with the clinician expertise and the patient's values and preferences, the best research evidence optimally informs clinical decisions. Because of the clinical reasoning and knowledge honed by APRNs, they are in the perfect position to provide leadership for integrating EBP into clinical practice,

---

Box 1
Components of knowledge management

1. Generating different types of evidence

2. Accumulating evidence to act as a repository

3. Synthesizing different forms of evidence

4. Translating evidence by evaluating, interpreting, and distilling

5. Disseminating evidence by formal and informal means

to serve as EBP mentors to other health care team members, and to communicate results by being a knowledge broker. If the APRN does not have the EBP competency suggested in this article, it is hoped that the processes for attaining these competencies have been delineated herein and could be incorporated into a personal action plan for future professional growth.

REFERENCES

1. Academic Center for Evidence-Based Practice (ACE); 2011. Available at: http://www.acestar.uthscsa.edu. Accessed October 25, 2011.
2. Stevens KR. ACE Star Model of EBP: Knowledge transformation. Academic Center for Evidence-Based Practice. The University of Texas Health Science Center at San Antonio; 2004. Available at: www.acestar.uthscsa.edu. Accessed October 25, 2011.
3. Moseley MJ. Establishing EBP performance competencies. Slide presentation from Second Annual 2003 Summer Institute on Evidence-Based Practice Best Practice: Improving Quality, 2003. Available at: http://www.acestar.uthscsa.edu/institute/su03/2003_Brochure/EBP.pdf. Accessed October 25, 2011.
4. Moseley MJ. Building an EBP team: Competencies & skill sets. Slide presentation from Third Annual 2004 Summer Institute on Evidence-Based Practice: Fostering Quality, 2004. Available at: http://www.acestar.uthscsa.edu/institute/su04/2004_brochure/811538%2004%20EBP.pdf. Accessed October 25, 2011.
5. Stevens KR. Essential competencies for evidence-based practice in nursing. 1st edition. San Antonio (TX): Academic Center for Evidence-Based Practice, UTHSCSA; 2005.
6. Grace J. Essential skills for evidence-based practice. How to ask a clinical question. J Nurs Sci 2009;27(1):1–10.
7. Strauss SE. Evidence-based medicine: how to practice and teach EBM. 3rd edition. Edinburgh (United Kingdom); New York: Elsevier/Churchill Livingstone; 2005.
8. University of Washington. Healthlinks; 2011. Available at: http://healthlinks.washington.edu/ebp/pico.html. Accessed October 25, 2011.
9. Centre for Evidence-Based Medicine Toronto. Formulating answerable clinical questions, 2011. Available at: http://ktclearinghouse.ca/cebm/practise/formulate/morepractise/therapy. Accessed October 25, 2011.
10. Slawson DC, Shaughnessy AF, Bennett JH. Becoming a medical information master: feeling good about not knowing everything. J Fam Pract 1994;38(5):505–13.
11. Siwek J, Gourlay ML, Slawson DC, et al. How to write an evidence-based clinical review article. Am Fam Physician 2002;65(2):251–8.
12. Booth A. Formulating answerable questions. In: Booth A, Brice A, editors. Evidence based practice for information professionals. London: Facet Publishing; 2004. p. 61–70.
13. Wildridge V, Bell L. How CLIP became ECLIPSE: A mnemonic to assist in searching for health policy/management information. Health Info Libr J 2002;19(2):113–5.
14. Sackett D, Richarson W, Rosenberg W, et al. Evidence-based medicine: how to practice and teach EBM. 1st edition. London: Elsevier; 1997.
15. Strauss SE, Richarson W, Glasziou Paul, et al. Evidence-based medicine: how to practice and teach EBM. 3rd edition. London: Elsevier; 2005.
16. Huang X, Lin J, Demner-Fushman D. Evaluation of PICO as a knowledge representation for clinical questions. AMIA Annu Symp Proc 2006;2006:359–63.

17. Kowalski K. The value of asking questions. J Contin Educ Nurs 2007;38(5):200.
18. Graner T, Sendelbach S, Boland LL, et al. Evidence-based nursing. Changing practice, one clinical question at a time. Nurs Manage 2011;42(5):14–7.
19. U.S. National Institutes of Health. 2011. PubMed. Available at: http://www.ncbi.nlm.nih.gov/pubmed/. Accessed October 27, 2011.
20. Majid S, Foo S, Luyt B, et al. Adopting evidence-based practice in clinical decision making: nurses' perceptions, knowledge, and barriers. J Med Libr Assoc 2011;99(3):229–36.
21. Newhouse RP, Stanik-Hutt J, White KM, et al. Advanced practice nurse outcomes 1990-2008: a systematic review. Nurs Econ 2011;29(5):1–21.
22. Duke University Medical Center Library & Health Sciences Library, UNC-Chapel Hill, 2010. Available at: Introduction to evidence based practice. http://www.hsl.unc.edu/Services/Tutorials/EBM/index.htm. Accessed October 27, 2011.
23. Buckingham J, Fisher B, Saunders D. Evidence based medicine toolkit, 2008. Available at: http://www.ebm.med.ualberta.ca/EbmIntro.html. Accessed October 27, 2011.
24. Katrak P, Bialocerkowski AE, Massy-Westropp N, et al. A systematic review of the content of critical appraisal tools. BMC Med Res Methodol 2004;4:22.
25. Sackett DL, Straus SE, Richardson WS, et al. Evidence-based medicine: how to practice and teach EBM. 2nd edition. London: Churchill Livingstone; 2000. p. 1.
26. Muller A, McCauley K, Harrington P, et al. Evidence-based practice implementation strategy: the central role of the clinical nurse specialist. Nurs Adm Q 2011;35(2):140–51.
27. Gerrish K, Guillaume L, Kirshbaum M, et al. Factors influencing the contribution of advanced practice nurses to promoting evidence-based practice among front-line nurses: findings from a cross-sectional survey. J Adv Nurs 2011;67(5):1079–90.
28. Gerrish K, McDonnell A, Nolan M, et al. The role of advanced practice nurses in knowledge brokering as a means of promoting evidence-based practice among clinical nurses. J Adv Nurs 2011;67(9):2004–14.

The Impact of Interprofessional Collaboration on the Effectiveness, Significance, and Future of Advanced Practice Registered Nurses

Dorothy Brooten, PhD, RN[a],*, JoAnne M. Youngblut, PhD, RN[b],
Jean Hannan, PhD, ARNP[b], Frank Guido-Sanz, MSN, ARNP[b]

KEYWORDS

- Interprofessional collaboration • Interprofessional education
- Interprofessional practice • Advanced practice registered nurse

KEY POINTS

- Advanced practice registered nurses (APRNs) improve care effectiveness and cost containment.
- Scope of practice of APRNs must expand in the future to meet health care needs.
- The nation's interprofessional collaboration is essential to achieve the goals of quality health care and reduced costs.

Growth in the numbers and roles of APRNs has occurred in the United States and globally.[1] This growth occurred because of a need for health care providers with advanced skills to meet an increase in demand for primary, preventive, and home care services, growing numbers of elders with complex health care needs, and increased patient acuity and complexity of hospital care. At present, implementation of the 2010 Affordable Health Care Act extends health coverage to an additional 32 million Americans by 2014[2] at a time of a predicted shortage of 40,000 primary care physicians. More than 250,000 APRNs (nurse practitioners, clinical nurse specialists, nurse midwives, and nurse anesthetists) are needed and well positioned to provide much of this care.[3] However, APRNs currently face barriers to providing such care because of restrictive state practice acts, restrictive prescriptive privileges, and opposition to expansion of

[a] Florida International University College of Nursing & Health Sciences, 11200 Southwest 8th Street, AHC III, Room 221, Miami, FL 33199, USA
[b] Florida International University College of Nursing & Health Sciences, 11200 Southwest 8th Street, Miami, FL 33199, USA
* Corresponding author.
E-mail address: Brooten@fiu.edu

Nurs Clin N Am 47 (2012) 283–294
doi:10.1016/j.cnur.2012.02.005
0029-6465/12/$ – see front matter © 2012 Elsevier Inc. All rights reserved.

their role from organized medical groups. For APRNs to succeed in providing a greater portion of the nation's health care and in expanding the APRN role, interdisciplinary collaboration is essential.

This article reviews issues on interdisciplinary collaboration that have been successfully addressed and those that challenge APRNs currently as they attempt to provide advanced care to the nation's citizens. In reviews of the literature, investigators have used the terms APNs and APRNs interchangeably. The term used by the original authors is used in this article.

INTERPROFESSIONAL COLLABORATION

The increasingly complex patient health problems being handled by health professionals are creating situations that demand more interdependence. Research has demonstrated that in settings where nurses collaborate as equals with other health care providers, patient outcomes and quality of care improve.[4] Interprofessional collaboration is key in initiatives to improve patient outcomes and to increase effectiveness of health services. Unfortunately, there is much diversity in conceptual definitions of interprofessional collaboration and the tools used to measure it.[5,6] Most definitions include elements of shared goals and partnerships, including explicit complementary and interdependent roles, mutual respect, and power sharing.[7] Power sharing is cited as one of the most complex aspects of interprofessional collaboration. As Rose[7] notes, ownership of specific knowledge, technical skills, clinical territory, or even the patient may produce interdisciplinary conflict.

Research shows that at a general level APNs and physicians agree on items needed for collaboration. However, APNs and clinicians think differently about behaviors needed for collaboration[8] and desirable traits of members of the other discipline.[9] Other studies indicate that nurses express more positive attitudes than physicians toward physician-nurse collaboration,[10] whereas other studies indicate that physicians report a higher degree of collaboration than do nurses.[11] Although some studies question the influence of gender on APN-physician collaboration, Rothstein and Hannum[12] report that the professionalism of the physician rather than gender plays a greater role. Other studies note the important role played by environments in fostering interprofessional collaboration, noting that fast-paced, interruptive environments reduce opportunities for communication and interpersonal relationships.[13,14] Others cite environmental barriers to interprofessional communication based on traditional hierarchal roles and responsibilities of physicians and nurses. Although collaboration implies interdependence as opposed to autonomy, much nursing literature is devoted to achievement of autonomy, which may be an inappropriate goal when striving for interdisciplinary collaboration.[7]

As the complexity of health care has increased, stakeholders are increasingly calling for health care professionals to work more collaboratively to provide care. Many have called for collaborative education for medical and nursing students, particularly in cultures with a hierarchical model of interprofessional relationships, to promote positive attitudes toward the complementary roles of physicians and nurses.[15] The need for faculty preparation in collaboration is recognized in such cultures before collaboration education can be carried out successfully.[10] Moreover, there may be a shortage of faculties prepared in interdisciplinary collaboration and interdisciplinary education. Some educators believe that interprofessional simulated learning experiences can be a valuable method of exploring shared leadership and collaborative ways of improving patient care and communication among health care professionals.[16] Other educators are skeptical of the lasting effects of interprofessional learning in the practice setting,[17] highlighting the need for interprofessional education to be integrated into experiences in clinical practice. The Institute of Medicine (IOM)[3] recommends that nurses be educated with physicians and other health professionals as students, and that interdisciplinary education and experiences occur throughout their careers. To date, there are limited reports of the outcomes of interprofessional education, and calls for rigorous studies in this area.[18]

The increasing complexity of health care, the growing demand for primary care services, and acceptance and expansion of the ARNP role require greater interprofessional collaboration. The support of interdisciplinary colleagues and other health care stakeholders has been and remains essential to the effectiveness, significance, and future contributions of ARNPs in the nation's health care.

INTERPROFESSIONAL COLLABORATION ON THE EFFECTIVENESS OF ARNPs

Establishing the effectiveness of ARNPs is essential in developing educational programs and standards, regulations, titling, prescribing privileges, and scope and standards of practice. Research has provided the evidence for ARNP effectiveness. Several hundred studies have been conducted examining APNs including outcomes of APN practices in primary care compared with physician practices,[19] acute care nurse practitioner (ACNP) hospital-managed care compared with that of physicians,[20] and research examining effects of APNs on patient outcomes and health care costs in vulnerable, high-volume, or high-cost patient groups.[21] Other research focused on the role of the APN, components of the role, time spent in each role component, and perceptions of the role by various stakeholders in health care. This research evolved through several stages: (1) research documenting effectiveness of ARNP practice compared with that of physicians to address issues of patient safety; (2) ARNPs working in extended roles with physician backup; (3) ARNPs working collaboratively with other health team members.

Studies in primary care comparing APN care with physician care have been conducted over several decades, and include high-volume patient groups such as women and children, elders, and those with chronic conditions.[19] Systematic reviews demonstrated that patients are more satisfied with APN care and that quality of care is equivalent or better than that of physicians.[22–26]

Studies in transitional care documented the effects of APN practice in improving patient outcomes and reducing health care costs.[21,27–32] In most of this research, APNs practiced in an expanded role with physician backup and consultation. As health care has become more complex, collaborative care by teams actively working together has become a necessity in improving outcomes, reducing health care costs, and providing better service delivery.[25,32,33]

The vast majority of studies documenting the effectiveness of APNs were conducted with nurses as principal investigators. However, because of the traditional roles and practices of APNs and physicians in health care systems, the studies required interdisciplinary collaboration. This collaboration was necessary because physicians served as gatekeepers in providing access to patients, discharging of patients, and controlling patient treatments. For major research funding, physician collaboration was required to document study access to patients. Physicians and members of other disciplines functioned as team members during the conduct of the studies, assisted in problem solving during the course of the studies, and were part of the teams in dissemination of study findings through publication and presentations. Without this level of interdisciplinary collaboration, many if not most of the studies documenting APN effectiveness in improving patient outcomes and reducing health care costs would not have occurred. Yet despite the numbers of studies demonstrating APN effectiveness, the translation of this effectiveness into shared goals, partnerships, acknowledgment of complementary and interdependent roles, mutual respect, and power sharing has lagged.

INTERPROFESSIONAL COLLABORATION ON THE SIGNIFICANCE OF ARNPs

In the United States, the nurse anesthetist was the earliest of the advanced practice roles, their history dates back to the late 1800s.[34] Although the nurse anesthetist role is acknowledged as the oldest advanced nursing specialty, it was not formalized until the twentieth century.[35] At present there are more than 44,000 Certified Registered Nurse Anesthetists (CRNAs) in practice in the United States in collaborative practices with physicians.[36]

The midwifery role was initially brought to the United States from England to fill a health care need in rural and underserved areas.[37] Integration of midwifery into professional nursing practice developed in the United States in the early 1900s. At present there are 18,492 Certified Nurse Midwives (CNMs) in practice in the United States,[38] practicing independently or collaboratively with physicians.

The Clinical Nurse Specialist (CNS) role, which developed in acute care settings and mental health hospital settings, has been established since 1954. In the 1960s master's programs for CNSs were developed, focusing on improving clinical care in hospitals and extended care facilities by coordinating care for patients, educating nursing personnel, and identifying and improving health care organizations.[38] Clinical specialty areas include, among others, oncology, pediatrics, geriatrics, psychiatric/mental health, adult health, and community health.[38] In 2008 there were an estimated 59,242 nurses prepared as CNSs, constituting the second largest group of APNs. Approximately 27% also had dual preparation in other advanced specialties such as dual CNS–nurse practitioner (NP).[38]

Establishment of the NP role dates to the late 1950s and the 1960s, when the need for primary care services in rural areas, for the underserved, low-income women, children, the elderly, and people with disabilities outstripped the ability of physicians to provide these services. With a nationwide shortage of physicians unable to meet this demand, physicians began mentoring and collaborating with nurses, and the NP role was established.[39] At present NPs make up the greatest numbers of APNs practicing in the United States. As of 2008 there were more than 158,000 NPs in the United States[38] and their numbers continue to grow. Their areas of specialty practice include community health nurse practitioner (CHNP), neonatal nurse practitioner (NNP), pediatric nurse practitioner (PNP), family nurse practitioner (FNP), adult nurse practitioner (ANP) and ACNP, among others. NPs work in independent practice or work collaboratively in physician practices.

In 1995 the role of the ACNP was developed.[40] ACNPs represent slightly more than 5% of the NPs practicing in the United States.[41] The role of ACNPs responded to an increased need for tertiary services and a shortage of physicians trained in intensive care. In intensive care units (ICUs), the role of ACNPs is evolving to replace physician care, and as a result[42] follows a medical model of care.[43] CNSs and NPs continue to be the predominant APNs in critical care units in the United States.[44] Differences in role definition and scope of practice of these 2 types of APNs are stipulated by their licensure and the governing state laws. In critical care, CNSs are more involved in case outcome, indirect care, and management, whereas ACNPs are more involved providing direct care,[44] which generates revenues.[40] ACNPs function as members of multidisciplinary teams in collaborative practice rather than individual or autonomous practice. Care provided by ACNPs has been documented in numerous studies examining quality of care,[20] morbidity, and mortality.[45-47] Results indicate that the quality of care provided by ACNPs is equal to that of physicians as well as being cost efficient.[24,48]

Initially NPs were viewed with suspicion and distrust by both nurses and physicians.[49] Many nurses viewed NPs as practicing medicine and no longer practicing nursing,[50] while physicians believed they would jeopardize the quality of medicine. NPs increased the availability of primary care services and research-documented patient and physician satisfaction with their quality of care.[51,52] In addition to providing services less expensively, NPs developed innovative health care models, which positioned them as health care reformers in efforts to provide high-quality health care services while controlling health care costs.

The classic work of Mundinger and colleagues[19] provided adult primary care services and admitting privileges for ARNPs, a model demonstrating quality patient outcomes, ARNP significance, partnership building, interdependent roles, mutual respect, and power sharing. To accomplish this required interdisciplinary collaboration from physicians and hospital administrators.

Other examples of innovative care models include NP-managed clinics and nurse-managed health centers (NMHCs). The more than 250 NMHCs in the United States serving an estimated 250,000 patients are largely independent nonprofit organizations or academically based clinics affiliated with schools of nursing.[53] These centers provide primary care, health promotion, and disease prevention services for the underserved, those living in poverty, the uninsured, or those with limited access to health care.[41] Care provided in NMHCs is cost effective and accessible, with outcomes similar to those of primary care physicians.[54,55] These clinics and NMHCs have collaborating physicians available to staff as salaried hires or as partners in the practice to meet state regulations.

Another model, the quality cost model of APN transitional care developed by Brooten and colleagues[27] and later modified by Naylor and colleagues,[32] provides comprehensive discharge planning and home follow-up to high-risk, high-volume, high-cost patient groups.[21] Results of clinical trials testing the model consistently documented improvements in patient outcomes and significantly reduced health care charges for the ARNP intervention groups.[21] Interdisciplinary collaboration from physicians and nurses was necessary for early discharge and home follow-up. The model, which demonstrated ARNP significance, interdependent roles, and mutual respect, is being recommended by stakeholders for inclusion under the Affordable Care Act.[56]

INTERPROFESSIONAL COLLABORATION ON THE FUTURE OF APNs

Several major initiatives, the Affordable Care Act, the consensus model, scope of practice (SOP) changes, and reimbursement for services, are essential to the future of ARNPs. All require interprofessional collaboration for success. Under the Affordable Care Act, health coverage will be extended to 32 million additional Americans by 2014.[2] This expansion is accompanied by a predicted shortage of 40,000 primary care physicians by 2020,[26] placing an immediate and future strain on the country's primary care system.[57,58]

The Affordable Care Act has important provisions for ARNPs, including: $50 million a year to establish graduate nurse education including programs for each of 4 ARNP roles; a mandatory funding stream for Title VIII programs including education grants to prepare the 4 types of ARNPs; a demonstration grant for a 1-year residency for NPs in federally qualified health centers and NMHCs; $50 million in grants for NMHCs; recognition of NPs and CNSs as "Accountable Care Organization (ACO) Professionals"; and

10% bonus payment under Medicare for primary care practitioners, including NPs and CNSs. In addition, the reimbursement rate for CNMs for covered services will be 100%, up from the previous rate of 65% compared with physician services.[59]

Establishing new or expanding existing NP clinics or NMHCs will increase access to care for millions of Americans.[38] This aspect is especially important because the elderly (older than 65 years) are a growing majority of people who will require a great deal of health care services. By 2030, there will be about 70 million older persons, making up 20% of the population, or 1 in 5 Americans.[38] Older adults are at higher risk for a variety of diseases compared with younger adults, and these diseases will occur with greater frequency among an older population. In 2007, about 12.9 million persons aged 65 and older accounted for short-stay hospital discharges, 3 times the rate for persons of all ages.[38] Older persons also averaged nearly half of all doctor visits. Almost 3% of elders failed to obtain needed medical care during the previous 12 months because of financial barriers.[38]

With reimbursement rates declining from Medicare and Medicaid, primary care providers are finding it increasingly difficult to keep their practices financially sustainable, and many are opting out of these government health care plans.[60] With the projected increase in elders, the shortage of health care providers, and practice limits on APNs, access to care for the elderly will become more difficult.

REIMBURSEMENT FOR APN SERVICES

NPs are challenged with obtaining adequate and reasonable reimbursement for the services they provide. Not only are they challenged with reduced reimbursement rates by Medicaid, but many private insurance companies do not recognize NPs as primary care providers. For the Affordable Care Act to achieve its goals, the IOM[3] recommends that state legislatures require that third-party payers in fee-for-service markets provide direct payment to NPs practicing within their SOP under state laws.

The United States Balanced Budget Act of 1997 resulted in reductions in federal Medicare spending.[61] Although the Act removed restrictions on geographic areas and settings in which NP services were reimbursed, it also resulted in NPs practicing independently of a physician to be reimbursed 85% of the physician fee schedule.[62] Medicare's 85% reimbursement rate is when care is provided without the direct supervision of a physician for the same health care services provided. A billing method for NPs to receive 100% reimbursement of the physician rate is known as incident to billing. In this method, services are billed under the physician's provider number when NPs provide services under the direct supervision of the physician. Regulations set by Medicare require that a physician must be physically present and immediately available to render assistance; the physician must conduct the initial visit and devise a care plan related to that episode of care.[53] Because many primary care facilities are struggling financially and depend on the 100% reimbursement rate, most practices prefer billing using the incident-to-billing reimbursement rate. This Medicare regulation promotes inefficient use of health care providers.[63] In addition, there are no studies reporting improved patient safety and improved outcomes when NPs provide care under physician supervision, compared with NP care without direct supervision.[3,64] However, studies documenting high-quality, cost-effective primary care provided by NPs, meeting the National Commission for Quality Assurance and Medicare Payment Advisory Commission standards of care for facilities such as NP-managed health centers, has not changed the incident-to-billing regulation.[41]

Medicaid does not follow the same NP reimbursement regulations as Medicare. Medicaid, a state-regulated program, varies in NP reimbursement regulations in each state. In 36 states, Medicaid is a fee-for-service plan that reimburses NPs directly at 100% of the physician rate, whereas other states reimburse NPs at a reduced rate.[57,58] In addition, federal law mandates that states reimburse family NPs and pediatric NPs for services provided to Medicaid patients, whereas other NPs (adult, geriatric) or NPs with other specialties are not included. This federal law, by not including reimbursement for adult, geriatric, or other NPs with specialty certification, is a limitation for Medicaid policy holders in their choice of providers. Thirty-six states that have recognized this as a barrier to care and have elected to reimburse all types of NPs, whereas other states continue to reimburse only pediatric NPs and family NPs.[65]

Other nonfederal third-party payers, such as commercial indemnity insurers, commercially managed care organizations/health maintenance organizations, and businesses or schools, often pay NPs at a lower rate than physicians for the same services or do not recognize NPs as primary a care provider.[66] A 2009 survey of 232 insurers conducted by National Nursing Centers Consortium[57,58] reported that nearly half (48%) of major managed care organizations credential NPs as primary care providers. Four percent of respondents stated that while they did not credential NPs as primary care providers, the NP services were provided to Medicaid beneficiaries or patients in rural areas where few primary care physicians exist. The report noted that state and federal laws designed to prohibit unfair discrimination continue to provide little protection for NPs. Such limitations on credentialing and reimbursement impede the ability of NPs to practice to the full scope of their education and training. However, more insurers are now allowing APNs to bill directly for their services, with some paying more than the 85% reimbursement rate for nurses compared with physician compensation for the same services.[67]

With federal health care reform resulting in millions of newly insured patients nationwide, NP-managed health centers, community health centers, and NP-led private practices are a key component of the nation's health care safety net. Because nearly half of all managed care organizations in the United States do not credential NMHCs as primary care providers, their capacity for growth and long-term sustainability is threatened.[57,58,68] Limiting the growth of these practices threatens implementation of the Affordable Care Act. With the limitations on NP practice, it is unclear whether the needs of a universally insured nation can be met unless it uses NPs as primary care providers. Without public recognition, nurse-led medical/health homes cannot qualify for insurance reimbursement, thus leaving substantial populations underserved, especially the indigent.[3]

CHANGES IN SCOPE OF PRACTICE

The 250,000 ARNPs with master's or doctoral degrees and who have passed national certification examinations are state regulated, providing care under the SOP provisions of the Nurse Practice Acts of their state. Because licensing and practice rules vary across states, regulations regarding SOP affect what ARNPs are allowed to do. Depending on the state, restrictions on NPs' SOP may limit or prohibit their authority to prescribe medications, admit patients to hospitals, assess patient conditions, and order and evaluate tests. Because the SOP varies among states, some NPs work independently of physicians, whereas in other states a collaborative agreement with a physician is required for practice.[63] The extent of the physician collaborative agreement, the role, duties, responsibilities, medical treatments, and pharmacologic prescriptions, among other practices, also varies widely among states. At present, 16 states plus the District of Columbia have expanded NP SOP regulations, allowing NPs to practice and prescribe independently.[2] Several states have granted NPs authority to prescribe controlled substances independently, but the majority of states allow this privilege only under a physician's supervision. While some states are currently evaluating their laws in efforts to expand NP SOP, most states continue to restrict NP practice.

With the potential implementation of the 2010 Affordable Care Act, interdisciplinary fights are becoming public. For physicians, dominance of their profession in providing health care is challenged.[69] Some physicians see reimbursement for ARNP services as an erosion of their earning potential.[67] The president of the American Society of Anesthesiologists stated concerns that physician oversight of health care will be compromised.[70] Physician groups are noting that if health care reform is pushing doctors' jobs into nurses' hands, it will only fuel resentment toward federal mandates.[70] The IOM,[3] however, wants nurses to gain more autonomy in practice and to take leadership roles on health care teams, including prescribing drugs and diagnosing disease with limited or no physician oversight, and is urging federal regulation to help achieve that goal. The report notes that primary care physicians and nurses tend to see cases of low or moderate complexity, and that there are no data on states with more restrictive SOP laws on what APNs can do demonstrating better quality outcomes in comparison with states with less restrictive laws. In addition, APN prescriptive practices are on a par with safety for physicians, that is, once established in practice ARNPs have the same rate of errors as physicians. The IOM report points out that the Federal Trade Commission has previously challenged anticompetitive policies and laws promulgated by the American Medical Association and state lawmakers on issues of physician supervision requirements and restrictions on nurse-run clinics. The IOM is urging federal agencies to design payment policies that encourage states to adopt up-to-date rules on nurses' practice.[70] With changes in the health care system over the years, there has been a growing acceptance on the part of state legislatures to expanded SOP for NPs; however, the power of medical organizations in resisting changes to nurse SOP can temper this acceptance. At present, organizations nationwide are working to develop ways to eliminate variations in SOP regulations across states.[3]

CONSENSUS MODEL

The Consensus Model for ARNP Regulation: Licensure, Accreditation, Certification & Education provides a model for future regulation of ARNPs and some critical agreement on education standards.[59] Work on the Model began in 2008 with planned implementation in 2015. Under the model, ARNPs would meet certain standardized education requirements including education in 1 of the 4 ARNP roles and in at least 1 population area (eg, family, adult-gerontology, women's health, neonatal, pediatrics, psychiatric–mental health). The ARNP core curriculum must include advanced physiology-pathophysiology, advanced health assessment, and advanced pharmacology. Under the model, licensing boards would no longer assess and regulate competency at the nursing specialty level. The boards would grant initial ARNP licensure based on ARNPs having graduated from an accredited program that prepared them in 1 of the 4 ARNP roles and in 1 population focus. Certification is recommended for specialty practice.[71] This model will help encourage the development of consistent regulations that recognize the competence of NPs across states.[2,3] It should also mute some arguments from medical organizations regarding ARNP education and regulation.

SUMMARY

If the 2010 Affordable Care Act is to be implemented in 2014, with all Americans having access to quality, affordable health care while containing health care costs, ARNPs will become essential to its implementation. ARNPs are the providers with the numbers and the expertise to do so, especially given the shortage of primary care physicians. However, as the IOM[3] has recommended, it is imperative that NPs are able to practice to the fullest extent of their education and training. To do so, all states need to allow ARNPs prescriptive authority regarding controlled substances and direct billing to Medicaid and insurance providers in the same manner and at the same rate as that of physicians. To accomplish this will require much continued interdisciplinary collaboration.

REFERENCES

1. Sheer B, Wong FK. The development of advanced nursing practice globally. J Nurs Scholarsh 2008;40(3):204–11.
2. Fairman JA, Rowe JW, Hassmiller S. Broadening the scope of nursing practice. N Engl J Med 2011;364(3):193–6.
3. The future of nursing: focus on scope of practice. Institute of Medicine; 2010. Available at: http://www.iom.edu/~/media/Files/Report%20Files/2010/The-Future-of-Nursing/Nursing%20Scope%20of%20Practice%202010%20Brief.pdf. Accessed October 23, 2011.
4. Naylor MD. Viewpoint: interprofessional collaboration and the future of health care. American Nurse Today, 6(6). Available at: http://www.americannursetoday.com/article.aspx?id=7908&fid=7870. Accessed October 26, 2011.
5. D'Amour D, Ferrada-Videla M, San Martin Rodriguez L, et al. The conceptual basis for interprofessional collaboration: core concepts and theoretical frameworks. J Interprof Care 2005;19(1):116–31.
6. Zwarenstein M, Goldman J, Reeves S. Interprofessional collaboration: effects of practice-based interventions on professional practice and healthcare outcomes. Cochrane Database Syst Rev 2009;3:CD000072.
7. Rose L. Interprofessional collaboration in the ICU: how to define? Nurs Crit Care 2011;16(1):5–10.
8. O'Brien JL, Martin DR, Heyworth JA, et al. A phenomenological perspective on advanced practice nurse-physician collaboration within an interdisciplinary healthcare team. J Am Acad Nurse Pract 2009;21(8):444–53.
9. Simpson KR, James DC, Knox GE. Nurse-physician communication during labor and birth: implications for patient safety. J Obstet Gynecol Neonatal Nurs 2006; 35(4):547–56.
10. Hojat M, Nasca TJ, Cohen MJ, et al. Attitudes toward physician-nurse collaboration: a cross-cultural study of male and female physicians and nurses in the United States and Mexico. Nurse Res 2001;50(2):123–8.
11. Copnell B, Johnston L, Harrison D, et al. Doctors' and nurses' perceptions of interdisciplinary collaboration in the NICU, and the impact of a neonatal nurse practitioner model of practice. J Clin Nurs 2004;13(1):105–13.
12. Rothstein WG, Hannum S. Profession and gender in relationships between advanced practice nurses and physicians. J Prof Nurs 2007;23(4):235–40.
13. Rice K, Zwarenstein M, Conn LG, et al. An intervention to improve interprofessional collaboration and communications: a comparative qualitative study. J Interprof Care 2010;24(4):350–61.
14. Weller JM, Barrow M, Gasquione S. Interprofessional collaboration among junior doctors and nurses in the hospital setting. Med Educ 2011;45(5):478–87.
15. Barrow M, McKimm J, Gasquione S. The policy and the practice: early career doctors and nurses as leaders and followers in the delivery of health care. Adv Health Sci Educ Theory Pract 2011;16(1):17–29.

16. Kenaszchuk C, MacMillan K, van Soeren M, et al. Interprofessional simulated learning: short-term associations between simulation and interprofessional collaboration. BMC Med 2011;9:29.
17. Murray-Davis B, Marshall M, Gordon F. What do midwives think about interprofessional working and learning? Midwifery 2011;27(3):376–81.
18. Reeves S, Zwarenstein M, Goldman J, et al. Interprofessional education: effects on professional practice and health care outcomes. Cochrane Database Syst Rev 2008;1:CD002213.
19. Mundinger MO, Kane RL, Lenz ER, et al. Primary care outcomes in patients treated by nurse practitioners or physicians. JAMA 2000;283(5):59–68.
20. Kleinpell R, Gawlinski A. Assessing outcomes in advanced practice nursing practice: the use of quality indicators and evidence-based practice. AACN Clin Issues 2005;16(1):43–57.
21. Brooten D, Naylor MD, York R, et al. Lessons learned from testing the quality cost model of Advanced Practice Nursing (APN) transitional care. J Nurs Scholarsh 2002;34(4):369–75.
22. Bauer CJ. Nurse practitioners as an underutilized resource for health reform: evidence-based demonstrations of cost-effectiveness. J Am Acad Nurse Pract 2010;22(4):228–31.
23. Bonsall K, Cheater FM. What is the impact of advanced primary care nursing roles on patients, nurses and their colleagues? A literature review. Int J Nurs Stud 2008;45(7):1090–102.
24. Horrocks S, Anderson E, Salisbury C. Systematic review of whether nurse practitioners working in primary care can provide equivalent care to doctors. BMJ 2002;6(324):819–23.
25. Kleinpell RM, Ely WE, Grabenkor R. Nurse practitioners and physician assistants in the intensive care unit: an evidence-based review. Crit Care Med 2008;36(10):2888–97.
26. Martin A. Nurse practitioners' growing role in your health care primary-care doctor shortage, health reform drives growth in NPs. Wall St J 2010. Available at: http://www.marketwatch.com/story/nurse-practitioners-growing-role-in-health-care-2010-06-02?pagenumber=1. Accessed October 23, 2011.
27. Brooten D, Kumar S, Brown L, et al. A randomized clinical trial of early discharge and home follow-up of very low birthweight infants. N Engl J Med 1986;315:934–9.
28. Brooten D, Roncoli M, Finkler S, et al. A randomized trial of early hospital discharge and home follow-up of women having cesarean birth. Obstet Gynecol 1994;84(5):832–8.
29. Brooten D, Youngblut JM, Brown L, et al. A randomized trial of nurse specialist home care for women with high risk pregnancies: outcomes and costs. Am J Manag Care 2001;7(8):793–803.
30. Naylor M, Brooten D, Jones R, et al. Comprehensive discharge planning for the hospitalized elderly: a randomized clinical trial. Ann Intern Med 1994;120(12):999–1006.
31. Naylor MD, Brooten D, Campbell R, et al. Comprehensive discharge planning and home follow-up of hospitalized elders: a randomized clinical trial. JAMA 1999;281:613–20.
32. Naylor MD, Brooten DA, Campbell RL, et al. Transitional care of older adults hospitalized with heart failure: a randomized, controlled trial. J Am Geriatr Soc 2004;52(5):675–84.
33. Cowan MJ, Shapiro M, Hays RD, et al. The effect of a multidisciplinary hospitalist/physician and advanced practice nurse collaboration on hospital costs. J Nurs Adm 2006;36(2):79–85.

34. Diers D. Nurse midwives and nurse anesthetists: the cutting edge in specialist practice. In: Aiken LH, Fagan CM, editors. Charting nursing's future: agenda for the 1990's. New York: Lippincott; 1991. p. 159–80.

35. Phillips SJ. 18th annual legislative update: a comprehensive look at the legislative issues affecting advanced nursing practice. Nurse Pract 2006;31(1):6–8, 11–7, 21–8.

36. American Association of Nurse Anesthetists. CRNA career center. Available at: http://www.aana.com/crnacareers.aspx. Accessed October 26, 2011.

37. Brucker M. History of midwifery. Parkland School of Nurse Midwifery history of midwifery in the US. Available at: http://www.neonatology.org/pdf/midwifery.history.pdf. Accessed October 23, 2011.

38. U.S. Department of Health and Human Services Health Resources Services Administration. The registered nurse population: Findings from the 2008 national sample survey of registered nurses. Available at: http://bhpr.hrsa.gov/healthworkforce/rnsurveys/rnsurveyfinal.pdf. Accessed October 25, 2011.

39. Division of Nursing, Bureau of Health Professions. The registered nurse population: findings from the national sample survey of registered nurses. Washington, DC: U.S. Department of Health and Human Services; 1996.

40. Cramer CL, Orlowski JP, DeNicola LK. Pediatric intensivist extenders in the pediatric ICU. Pediatr Clin North Am 2008;55(3):687–708.

41. American Academy of Nurse Practitioners. Nurse practitioner facts. Available at: http://www.aanp.org/NR/rdonlyres/54B71B02-D4DB-4A53-9FA6-23DDA0EDD6FC/0/NPFacts2010.pdf. Accessed October 22, 2011.

42. Knaus VL, Felten S, Burton S, et al. The use of nurse practitioners in the acute care setting. J Nurs Adm 1997;27(2):20–7.

43. Irvine D, Sidani S, Porter H, et al. Organizational factors influencing nurse practitioners' role implementation in acute care settings. Can J Nurs Leadersh 2000;13(3):28–35.

44. Coombs M, Chaboyer W, Sole ML. Advanced nursing roles in critical care—a natural or forced evolution? J Prof Nurs 2007;23(2):83–90.

45. Hoffman LA, Tasota FJ, Zullo TG, et al. Outcomes of care managed by an acute care nurse practitioner/attending physician team in a subacute medical intensive care unit. Am J Crit Care 2005;14(2):121–30.

46. Meyer SC, Miers LJ. Cardiovascular surgeon and acute care nurse practitioner: collaboration on postoperative outcomes. AACN Clin Issues 2005;16(2):149–58.

47. Munro N, Taylor-Panek S. The nurse practitioner role: the communication link for cardiac surgery patients. Crit Care Nurs Clin North Am 2007;19(4):385–94.

48. Kinnersley P, Anderson E, Parry K, et al. Randomised controlled trial of nurse practitioner versus general practitioner care for patients requesting "same day" consultations in primary care. BMJ 2000;320(7241):1043–8.

49. O'Brien JM. How nurse practitioners obtained provider status: lessons for pharmacists. Am J Health Syst Pharm 2003;60(22):2301–7.

50. Nichols BL. Nurse practitioners: the American experience. Wis Med J 1997;96(6):16–8.

51. Mendenhall RC, Repicky PA, Neville RE. Assessing the utilization and productivity of nurse practitioners and physician's assistants: methodology and findings on productivity. Med Care 1980;18(6):609–23.

52. Record JC, McCally M, Schweitzer SO, et al. New health professions after a decade and a half: delegation, productivity, and costs in primary care. J Health Polit Policy Law 1980;5(3):470–97.

53. American College of Physicians. Nurse practitioners in primary care. A policy monograph of the American College of Physicians. Available at: http://www.acponline.org/advocacy/where_we_stand/policy/np_pc.pdf. Accessed October 23, 2011.

54. Barkauskas VH, Pohl JM, Tanner C, et al. Quality of care in nurse-managed health centers. Nurs Adm Q 2011;35(1):34–43.
55. Hansen-Turton T, Line L, O'Connell M, et al. The nursing center model of health care for the underserved (HCFA Contract No. 18–P91720/3-01). Philadelphia: National Nursing Centers Consortium; 2004.
56. Naylor MD, Aiken LH, Kurtzman ET, et al. The care span: the importance of transitional care in achieving health reform. Health Aff (Millwood) 2011;30(4):746–54.
57. National Nursing Centers Consortium. The nurse-managed health clinic investment act of 2007 (S.112). Available at: http://www.nncc.us/policy/NMHCAct.pdf. Accessed August 25, 2008.
58. National Nursing Centers Consortium. Nurse-managed health centers. Available at: http://www.nncc.us/site/pdf/NNCC%20-%20Health%20Center%20FS%202009.pdf. Accessed October 21, 2011.
59. Summers L. How the health care reform law affects APRNs. Am Nurse 2010; 42(3):16.
60. Siegel M. When doctors opt out: we already know what government-run health care looks like. Wall Street Journal 2009. Available at: http://online.wsj.com/article/SB123993462778328019.html. Accessed October 25, 2011.
61. Schneider A. Overview of Medicaid provisions in the Balanced Budget Act of 1997, P.L. 105-33. Center on Budget and Policy Priorities. Available at: http://www.cbpp.org/cms/index.cfm?fa=view&id=2138. Accessed October 20, 2011.
62. The Kaiser commission on Medicaid and the uninsured. Kaiser Family Foundation; 2011. Available at: www.kff.org. Accessed October 25, 2011.
63. Dower C, Christian S, O'Neil E. Promising scope of practice models for the health professions. San Francisco (CA): Center for the Health Professions University of California. Available at: http://chpe.creighton.edu/events/roundtables/2009-2010/pdf/scope.pdf. Accessed October 23, 2011.
64. Center to Champion Nursing in America. Access to care and advanced practice nurses: a review of Southern U.S. Practice Laws. Washington, DC: AARP Public Policy Institute; 2010. Available at: http://www.achi.net/HCR%20Docs/2011HCR WorkforceResources/Access%20to%20Care%20APNs.pdf. Accessed October 23, 2011.
65. Phillips SJ. 22nd Annual legislative update: regulatory and legislative successes for APNs. Nurse Pract 2010;35(1):24–47.
66. Buppert C. Nurse practitioner's business practice and legal guide. 3rd edition. Massachusetts: Jones and Bartlett; 2008. p. 5.
67. McNamara M. Nurse practitioners' role as primary care providers sparks debate. Am Nurse 2010;42(3):14.
68. Hansen-Turton T. New research shows that insurer contracting policies threaten success of health care reform. Public Health Management Corporation; 2009 [press release]. Available at: http://www.phmc.org/site/index.php?option=com_content&view=article&id=371:new-research-shows-that-insurer-contracting-policies-threaten-success-of-health-care-reform&catid=45:2009&Itemid=1574. Accessed October 23, 2011.
69. Gardner D. Expanding scope of practice: inter-professional collaboration or conflict? Nurs Econ 2010;28(4):264–6.
70. Carlson J. Fueling the turf battle. Institute of Medicine report pushes expanded scope for nurses; docs say study draws illogical conclusions. Mod Healthc 2010;40(41):6–7, 16, 1.
71. Trossman S. Coming together to secure strong future for APRNs. Am Nurse 2008; 40(4):1, 8–9, 18.

The Future of the Psychiatric Mental Health Clinical Nurse Specialist: Evolution or Extinction

Anita Dempsey, PhD, APRN, PMHCNS-BC[a],*, Judy Ribak, PhD, APRN, PMHCNS-BC[b]

KEYWORDS

- Psychiatric clinical nurse specialist • Certification • Future role
- Advanced practice registered nurse

KEY POINTS

- The psychiatric mental health clinical nurse specialist (PMHCNS) was the first clinical nurse group to establish specialty certification.
- The role of the PMHCNS includes education in social and psychological models, theory, and individual and group psychotherapeutic treatment methods necessary for comprehensive treatment.
- Although the PMHCNS certification examination will be retired in 2014, other groups can be brought into a similar role through mentoring or expanding the scope of practice.

The role of the psychiatric mental health clinical nurse specialist (PMHCNS) is now in a precarious position. At first glance, some may say it is on the verge of extinction. Because fewer individuals select the specialty option of PMHCNS and in an attempt of the American Nurses Credentialing Center (ANCC) to support the Consensus Model for advanced practice registered nurse (APRN) regulation recommendations (2008),[1] the ANCC has announced that as of 2014 the certification examination for the PMHCNS will be retired.[2] Those currently holding PMHCNS certification have been assured of the ability to continue to practice in the PMHCNS advanced role, as long as all certification renewal requirements regarding professional development activities and clinical practice hours are met in accordance with individual state licensure requirements. However, any lapse in certification may result in the loss of ability to renew certification and, subsequently, the license to practice as an APRN.[2] This is an alarming message to the PMHCNS, and it certainly indicates a change for this advanced practice nursing role. This change will most certainly lead to the eventual extinction of the originally conceived and currently practiced PMHCNS. As we prepare to implement this sweeping

[a] College of Nursing and Health, Wright State University, 3640 Colonel Glenn Highway, Dayton, OH 45435-0001, USA
[b] Wright State University, College of Nursing and Health, Dayton, OH, USA
* 7660 Burlinehills Court, Cincinnati, OH 45244.
E-mail address: anita.dempsey@wright.edu

Nurs Clin N Am 47 (2012) 295–304
doi:10.1016/j.cnur.2012.02.003   **nursing.theclinics.com**

change, it is crucial that the role of the PMHCNS be fully understood so that critical functions do not fall by the wayside. In this article, a brief history of the role of the PMHCNS is reviewed along with current education, practice, role, and ANCC certification of the PMHCNS. The future implications and considerations of the unique functions of the PMHCNS for an APRN with a psychiatric mental health specialization are discussed.

HISTORY

Historically, psychiatric/mental health nurses have been nursing leaders and entrepreneurs. Psychiatric/mental health nurses, in the 1950s, recognized the need for educational and clinical criteria to function as a clinical nurse specialist (CNS), and were the first clinical nursing group to establish certification at the specialist level.[3] The scope of education and practice for the PMHCNS included social and psychological models; a variety of theoretical frameworks to facilitate the understanding of individuals, groups, and systems; and a variety of individual and group psychotherapeutic treatment modalities to support comprehensive treatment and consultation. During the 1980s, an influx of newly prepared CNSs, eager to practice in specialty areas, provided expert clinical care in acute and private settings, consultation services, staff and consumer education, and clinical leadership, and participated in the generation of evidence as a means to achieve the goal of improved outcomes of patient care. Advanced practice nurses, engaged in the role of the PMHCNS, contributed considerably to the quality and continuity of care for patients and family systems in both inpatient and outpatient practice settings. The aim of the PMHCNS has always been to assist the patient to achieve the highest possible level of wellness.

As the role of the PMHCNS emerged, each practitioner modeled the role within the parameters of traditional areas of practice with attention to the needs of the organization and environment of patient care. The PMHCNS became a valued resource providing education, clinical supervision, and mentoring for staff nurses as well as for other professionals within the environment of patient care. Over a period, PMHCNS roles were implemented and interpreted by those who fulfilled the roles to include focus on the treatment of individuals with complex mental health problems, often superimposed upon by both physical health problems and overwhelming psychosocial concerns. The PMHCNS provided the patient (and family) the increased time, attention, and support that physicians did not provide because the physician's traditional focus had been the patient's chief complaint or acute health problem at hand. The PMHCNS was the professional group that forged therapeutic relationships and helped form alliances with individuals and families who needed holistic care to both treat the acute health problem and intervene to address the accompanying psychosocial concern. The PMHCNS had very efficiently developed an independent and complementary role in the treatment of individuals with complex mental health problems, not as a physician extender, but as a holistic care provider with a nursing perspective.

Peplau[4] was clairvoyant in her assumption that the CNS could achieve expertise in the care of individuals with complex health concerns, and in treating the individual and family from a nursing perspective as opposed to the care offered by traditional medicine. Practicing alongside other mental health professionals, in all health care venues, the PMHCNS became the go-to practitioner for expert clinical care, consultation, education, clinical leadership, and research activities. The broad knowledge base, which integrated the physical with the psychosocial, provided a unique and valuable perspective to members of mental health treatment teams as well as to health care system administrators struggling to maintain quality in the rapidly changing health care environment.

CURRENT CNS PRACTICE AND PREPARATION

According to the 2009 Role Delineation Study, there are currently an estimated 6624 PMHCNSs.[5] At the time of the survey, 65% of the participants were 55 years or older, 90% had 20 or more years of experience as a registered nurse, and 80% had been certified as a PMHCNS for 10 or more years.[6] Thus, current PMHCNSs appear to be an older group with a lot of experience. However, as noted in the 2009 Role Delineation Study,[5,6] there has been a decline in individuals taking the PMHCNS certification examination. In 2010, a total of 82 individuals passed the ANCC adult psychiatric mental health certification examination. By contrast, 302 individuals passed the family psychiatric and mental health nurse practitioner (FPMHNP) certification, and 384 individuals passed the adult psychiatric mental health nurse practitioner certification.[6]

The current PMHCNS is the clinical expert at the advanced practice level of care. Inseparable and embedded in the current role are all the functions as originally indicated by the PMHCNS preparation. The PMHCNS is a practitioner who not only defines the diagnosis but also uses multiple modalities to provide patient care, practicing in specialty areas to provide expert clinical care including medication, psychotherapy, consultation services, staff and consumer education, clinical leadership, and generation of evidence. Consider the role of the PMHCNS in the following case.

The patient was an 86-year-old woman, living alone, who had fallen in her home. She had 3 grown-up children, living out of town, who were busy with careers and families of their own. One of the daughters was unable to reach her mother on the phone for 24 hours, and became worried, so she phoned the neighbor who went over to look in on the patient. The patient had been down for at least 10 hours. After an evaluation by the emergency department, the patient had been hospitalized in a senior adult mental health unit, with change in mental status, weight loss, gait disturbance, and possible dysphagia. Two of the daughters came to their mother's side within hours. They were both quite concerned that there had been a dramatic decline in their mother's condition since their most recent visit 4 months ago. Although the patient was glad to see both daughters, there had certainly been a memory decline, difficulty in finding words, and dramatic weight loss.

The PMHCNS met with the patient to complete a baseline evaluation of mental status as well as to obtain the history, current health problems, medication profile, and patient's perception of the current problem. The PMHCNS then met with the daughters to ascertain some of the same information, realizing that the daughters did not have daily or immediate contact with their mother. The PMHCNS investigated current health problems, medications, and treatments with the primary care physician. The gait disturbance was neither reported nor treated previously, and there was also no previously documented concern of confusion in this patient.

The PMHCNS made daily rounds to reassess the patient as well as to keep current on her hospital course, including multidisciplinary assessments and treatments, laboratory results, and diagnostic testing. The patient was found to have global cognitive loss as well as associated gait disturbance and dysphagia. After consultation with the unit nursing staff, occupational therapist, primary care physician, psychiatrist, gastroenterologist, physical therapist, and speech therapist, the PMHCNS prepared a comprehensive report including potential paths for the continued care of the patient.

The primary care physician recommended assisted living; the physical therapist recommended use of a walker and a structured exercise program; the psychiatrist recommended adding an antidepressant; the speech therapist recommended thickening liquids to increase safety in swallowing; the occupational therapist recommended structured recreational activity; and the gastroenterologist recommended permanent insertion of a gastrointestinal tube to provide nutrition, which would eliminate the possibility of aspiration when feeding by mouth.

The PMHCNS called a family meeting and invited the professionals as well as the patient and her children. The patient and her daughters were anxious to hear recommendations for restoring the good health that the patient had enjoyed nearly all her life. The family meeting was conducted by the PMHCNS, who began by exploring with the daughters the changes they found in their mother just before this admission. Each specialist (who attended) presented assessment findings and recommendations for the patient; the CNS then aptly explained the findings of those who were not present, in addition to the psychiatric findings, and invited questions.

The daughters were pleased by the recommendations of each specialist and were eager to proceed with every recommendation on their mother's behalf. The patient, however, was not very pleased about all the changes, including the recommendation to shift her residence and insert a feeding tube. "But mother, as soon as you accept these recommendations, you will feel better again, you will be walking more safely, and you will be back to your old self!" her daughter exclaimed.

The PMHCNS, alerted by the false promise that "you will be back to your old self," asks the daughter to elaborate. The CNS is an expert in providing care and is also alert to unspoken messages communicated in meeting with families, readily able to correct misperceptions and provide in-depth explanation. The feeding tube, for example, would not prevent all aspiration, though it would prevent aspiration from oral intake. The gait disorder would not be resolved by implementation of the exercises and walker; however, the patient would be safer only if she used the assistive device appropriately. There are implications when shifting the residence of a frail individual; the CNS addressed these implications as well. Group psychotherapy skills were used during this meeting; consultation with the family occurred on an ongoing basis during every step of the hospitalization; the multidisciplinary staff was apprised of the patient's and family's course during the hospitalization; clinical leadership was demonstrated as the CNS modeled communication with the patient, family, and multidisciplinary team. The CNS debriefed the nursing staff regarding this patient's care because the patient's primary care nurse was upset at the notion of placing a feeding tube. "Why can't they simply allow her to eat, if she enjoys food?" the distressed staff nurse asked. The CNS provided support for the nurse's concerns, because she used evidence to demonstrate the signs of dysphagia on using the feeding tube. "You are so correct, evidence supports that a patient may continue to aspirate despite insertion of a feeding tube, and the patient and her family now understand this," the CNS replied.

This simulated case demonstrates the expanded practice role that the PMHCNS implements every day. Debriefing the staff regarding the care of the patient, care of families facing the changing health of a member, and interpretation of the tests and procedures are all within the purview of the CNS. The comprehensive nature of care represented by this patient's experiences represents the relationships and roles of the PMHCNS. The role is crucial to both exemplary patient/family care as well as model communication among the disciplines.

Despite the ability to manage complex patient/family situations and to work with a variety of professionals, the ANCC certification criteria for a PMHCNS are the least rigorous when viewed alongside the ANCC certification criteria for the psychiatric and Mental Hhealth Nnurse Ppractitioner (PMHNP) and FPMHNP. Although the PMHCNS criteria were the first developed, they do not seem to fully reflect the many facets of the PMHCNS role. The requirement for the PMHCNS to have education regarding health promotion, disease prevention, differential diagnosis, and disease management is not specified. These functions, however, have for several years been a part of the PMHCNS role and educational curricula. All roles require a minimum of 500 super-vised clinical hours and clinical training in 2 psychotherapeutic specialties. It is clear in hindsight that the current PMHCNS certification did not reflect, and currently does not reflect, the scope, skills, knowledge, and value of the historical role of the PMHCNS. Although at first glance there appear to be equal clinical requirements for these 3 certifications, it is worth pointing out that the broader the scope of practice, the more content the 500 supervised clinical hours needs to cover. Thus, the PMHCNS has a more focused clinical experience on aspects of psychiatric mental health in the CNS role, including direct patient care with individuals and families, staff development, clinical supervision, research activities, group facilitation, and consultation, in addition to organizational and systems issues. The PMHNP is focused on providing physical and mental health care to the individual whereas the FPMHNP is focused on providing physical and mental health care to the individual and family, irrespective of age. The broader the clinical scope, the narrower the clinical focus that is concentrated on psychiatric mental health.

The education to become a PMHCNS shows a great degree of variability and flux. While these programs prepare one for practice, they must also prepare one to meet the ANCC certification requirements. A review of a limited sample of study programs that prepare advanced practice nurses for the PMHCNS or PMHNP role (**Table 1**) shows great variability in how these roles are conceptualized. Several individuals iden-tify the role of the PMHCNS as different from that of the PMHNP, by virtue of the focus of the PMHNP on provision of direct patient care, including prescription of medication and interpretation of diagnostic testing. Psychotherapy, a part of the PMHCNS role, is not necessarily seen to be within the scope of the PMHNP practice by some, but is seen to be so by others. Other than for direct patient care, there is little description to support multiple practice roles in the current role of the PMHNP. Collaborative, mentoring, group-facilitating, and interdisciplinary roles are not clearly defined by the PMHNP by program descriptions. Contrary to what the CNS role defines, the PMHNP role does not emphasize care of the family or case management. Clinical supervision of clinical providers is not an indicated skill of the PMHNP, although it is critical for the PMHCNS to be proficient at this skill. There is often minimal difference between the curricula of the PMHCNS and PMHNP study programs. One might assume that the difference is in the clinical experience; however, this is not consistently or clearly specified. Some univer-sity settings have suspended admissions to their master's level PMHCNS (and other CNS) programs, referring interested applicants to pursue CNS education at the doctoral level of education in the form of the doctorate of nursing practice (DNP) programs.

THE PMHCNS AND THE CONSENSUS MODEL

Some may have thought that the Consensus Model was simply another white paper written with thoughts and aspirations of a professional body wanting a seat at the adult table. It is clear that many other professions have already realigned their professional degrees to include doctoral level for the clinical expert degrees, that is, doctor of psychology, doctor of pharmacy, doctor of audiology, and doctor of physical therapy. The Consensus Model recommendations are vaguely reminiscent of the 1985 entry into practice proposal that mandated a dramatic philosophic shift regarding basic nursing education.[12] The realization that the entry into practice proposition was never

Table 1
A sample of 5 programs of study for the PMHCNS and NP

Educational Program	NP	CNS
The Ohio State University[7]	"Theoretical and evidence-based clinical knowledge that is essential for comprehensive primary care and specialty practice in a variety of settings"[7] "Diagnose and manage acute episodic and long-term illnesses and emphasize health promotion, illness prevention, and interprofessional collaboration"[7]	"Expert in diagnosis, treatment, remediation and alleviation of illnesses and to promote health within a specialty population"[7] "Provides highly specialized nursing care, serves as the clinical nursing expert for a unit or service line; and also implements the role for clinical coordinator, case manager, staff and patient educator and participant in research projects"[7]
University of California, San Francisco[8] Psychiatric/Mental Health Nursing "Advanced practice psychiatric nurses provide comprehensive patient-centered mental health care to individuals, groups, and families across the lifespan. An advanced practice psychiatric nurse may function as a Clinical Nurse Specialist, Nurse Practitioner or, in some cases, both"[8]	"Primary mental health care services including biopsychosocial assessment and diagnosis of patients with mental illness. Treatment modalities include both medication and psychotherapeutic management"[8]	"Incorporates research, clinical leadership, education, consultation, and expert clinical practice. Expert PMHCNS practice includes provision of psychotherapy"[8]
Vanderbilt University	"Assess, diagnose, plan, implement, intervene, manage and evaluate holistic plans of care—including treatment with psychotropic medications; individual, group and family psychotherapy; crisis intervention; case management and consultation"[9]	No program offered

University of Pittsburgh	"Prepared as a principal provider of primary health care who manages the care of adult psychiatric clients in a variety of settings on both an episodic and continuous basis"[10]	"Care of patients with psychiatric or psychosocial issues, including the delivery of psychotherapy. Nurses are prepared to be therapists, consultants, mental health educators, case managers, and supervisors"[a,10]
Indiana University Advanced Practice Psychiatric Mental Health Nurse. The program prepares the student to sit for PMHCNS or PMHNP certification examination[11]	"Designed to prepare graduate students in the diagnosis, treatment, and prevention of mental illness. The program also prepares students in case management, professional leadership, and interdisciplinary collaboration across a wide range of health care settings"[11]	"Designed to prepare graduate students in the diagnosis, treatment, and prevention of mental illness. The program also prepares students in case management, professional leadership, and interdisciplinary collaboration across a wide range of health care settings"[11]

Data retrieved from the identified school of nursing's current Web site as specified in the reference list.

Abbreviation: NP, nurse practitioner.

[a] MSN program applications suspended as of June 2011 in favor of the doctorate of nursing practice program for CNS education.

implemented and the divisiveness that has since haunted our profession for years after have been quite a dose to swallow. Years of hard work and discussion preceded its appearance, but every stakeholder group would not buy in, and there was ultimately enough dissent to stop the proposition from ever becoming a reality, no matter how noble the cause. The move to provide consistent definitions and points of entry into advanced nursing practice is ambitious and necessary to move advanced practice nursing forward in a deliberate and thoughtful manner.

The Consensus Model for APRN regulation (2008) provides comprehensive definitions for the CNS and the certified nurse practitioner (CNP) along with the minimal educational requirements necessary for certification and entry on licensure into advanced nursing practice. The Consensus Model defines the CNP as one prepared to deliver expert care to the individual or family system in his or her area of practice expertise. The CNS fulfills this care function for individuals and families in addition to working within systems mentoring, facilitating change and evidenced-based practice. In addition to participating in the generation and use of evidence in nursing science, the PMHCNS is a provider of expert clinical care, consultation services, staff and consumer education, and clinical leadership. The PMHCNS acts as a mentor to nurse generalists and beginning APRNs, and provides clinical supervision to members of health care teams. Yet these skills are not clearly reflected by the ANCC certification and, as the role is slated for retirement, these skills are in danger of being lost. Given the scope of the PMHCNS and its broad responsibilities in an increasingly complex and evolving health care environment, it is imperative that the skills and functions that the PMHCNS has brought to the mental health table not be lost as the PMHCNS certification is retired. Those expert clinical, organizational, and mentoring skills must be preserved.

For a newly educated APRN interested in providing psychiatric and mental health nursing care, the FPMHNP will become the certification credential for entry into advanced mental health nursing practice, because the PMHCNS and PMHNP retires in 2014.[13] Therefore, the generality of specialty-focused designations becomes apparent as the current population and specialty designations collapse into fewer numbers, and this collapse will accurately reflect on the generalist's entry into advanced practice.

Mind the Gaps

Although the Consensus Model for APRN regulation articulates the CNS role, the foundational educational requirement for advanced practice nurses offers only vague direction regarding the educational requirements for the CNS. This vagueness is frequently reflected in the master's level curricula, in which there is minimal difference between the CNS and nurse practitioner (NP) curricula. Given the broader scope of CNS practice and the need for specialty expertise, the American Association of Colleges of Nursing recommendation for advanced nursing practice preparation to be at the doctoral level and the shift in several nursing programs in moving their CNS programs to a doctoral level seems appropriate. The DNP offers the educational venue for advanced NPs in the role of CNS to gain specialized knowledge that extends beyond the direct focus of the NP on patient care. The DNP with a specialty in psychiatric and mental health nursing is the logical next step. Although work on the practice doctorate began years ago, and thoughtful development and discussion of purpose and curricula have since ensued, the PMHCNS needs to be at the table as these discussions continue.

Another difficulty in the current interpretation of the Consensus Model lies in the absence of statements that would directly address some critical elements of the

PMHCNS (see **Table 1**). Apparent in this discovery is the notion that several roles of the PMHCNS do not consistently appear in writing within current curricula or within the ANCC certification requirements for roles incorporating psychiatric mental health care, even though these roles will undoubtedly continue to be practiced by those who retain the PMHCNS designation. The roles include education and mentoring of nurses who provide psychiatric and mental health care, clinical supervision, debriefing, facilitating system changes, supporting development and use of evidence-based approaches aimed at improving nursing care, promoting improved clinical outcomes for psychiatric and mental health patients and their families, facilitating ethical decision making, and promoting diversity.

MOVING FORWARD

The role of the PMHCNS is at a crossroads: evolution or extinction. Although advanced practice roles may be maintained, ranks are dwindling and the ANCC certification examination is slated to be retired in 2014. The future of the PMHCNS, for those certified before 2014, requires vigilance to continue educational development and clinical practice and to maintain the advanced practice nursing credential and role. After 2014, when the PMHCNS certification will no longer be available, the ranks, as currently defined through certification, will continue to dwindle by attrition. The current PMHCNS certification will thus become extinct; however, the role can survive. This is not the time for complacency. We are challenged to educate others on the role and to demonstrate the value that the PMHCNS brings to the patient, family, multidisciplinary team, organization, community, and profession. Nursing practice has evolved over the years to become the most available profession for the patient. The nurse is the professional who spends most time with the patient and family, who knows the intricacies of the family, who has connected with the family unit in a way that other health professionals have not had the opportunity to, and is truly able to provide holistic care to the individual and the family. The challenge for the PMHCNS is to clearly demonstrate and communicate the comprehensive role that incorporates the mental health care of patient and family systems as well as the nursing and health care systems. Knowledge of physical, psychological, and social systems, and how they interact, allows for unique patient views and world views that guide our practice.

As PMHCNSs, we need to mentor nurses in mental health areas as well as throughout patient care systems to address the psychiatric mental health needs of patients in whatever setting they present. The PMHCNS is the consultant to mental health nursing staff and nurses in other general and specialty areas regarding care of the individual with mental health issues and needs. While institutions of higher learning evolve curricula for the newly devised advanced practice professional, nursing needs to pledge not to give up roles within patient care that are best delivered by the PMHCNS. We need to be actively involved in development of the evolving DNP with a specialty in psychiatric mental health nursing, to ensure that nurses remain at the table with other mental health professionals, as credible skilled clinicians offering unique holistic views and able to create and use evidence to guide practice.

Although the title may be retained, the scope of practice is more important. We must not be content to wait for change to arrive. We must be an active part of the evolution that is occurring if our role is to survive. Drawing on the examples of the psychiatric nursing leaders who have paved the way, it is up to us to be actively involved in this changing world. With a broad scope of specialty practice, the PMHCNS is well suited to continue implementing this role. The PMHCNS has a voice and it must be used. We are challenged to explore, advise, and advocate as to how the unique qualities of the PMHCNS, which are in jeopardy of extinction, can be integrated into advanced practice psychiatric mental health nursing education and practice as it continues to develop. Looking toward the future, it is up to the PMHCNS to ensure that the ability to provide a variety of psychiatric and mental health treatment modalities is maintained, so that the advanced practice nurse can continue to address psychiatric and mental health needs holistically, across settings and across the health care continuum.

REFERENCES

1. APRN Joint Dialogue Group Report, 2008. Consensus Model for APRN regulation: licensure, accreditation, certification and education. Available at: www.aacn.nche.edu/Education/pdf/APRNReport.pdf. Accessed November 14, 2011.
2. American Nurses Credentialing Center (ANCC), 2011. Consensus Model for APRN regulations, frequently asked questions. Available at: http://www.nursecredentialing.org/APRN-FAQ.aspx. Accessed October 28, 2011.
3. Critchley DL, Maurin JT. The clinical nurse specialist in psychiatric mental health nursing. New York: John Wiley and Sons; 1985.
4. Peplau H. Specialization in professional nursing. Nurs Sci 1965;3:268.
5. American Nurses Credentialing Center (ANCC), 2010. 2009 Role delineation study: clinical nurse specialist in adult psychiatric and mental health nursing—national survey results. Available at: http://www.nursecredentialing.org/Documents/Certification/RDS/2009RDSSurveys/AdultPsychCNS-2009RDS.aspx. Accessed November 1, 2011.
6. American Nurses Credentialing Center (ANCC), 2010. 2010 ANCC certification statistics. Available at: http://www.nursecredentialing.org/Certification/FacultyEducators/Statistics.aspx. Accessed November 1, 2011.
7. The Ohio State University School of Nursing (OSU). Available at: http://nursing.osu.edu/Display.aspx?code=141. Accessed November 21, 2011.
8. University of California San Francisco School of Nursing (UCSF). Available at: http://nursing.ucsf.edu/programs/specialties/psychiatricmental-health-nursing. Accessed November 21, 2011.
9. Vanderbilt University School of Nursing (UV). Available at: http://www.nursing.vanderbilt.edu/msn/pmhnp_plan.html. Accessed November 21, 2011.
10. University of Pittsburgh: School of Nursing (UP). Available at: http://www.nursing.pitt.edu/academics/masters/clinical.jsp. Accessed November 21, 2011.
11. Indiana University School of Nursing. Available at: http://nursing.iupui.edu/. Accessed November 21, 2011.
12. Christy TE. A recurring issue in nursing history. Lippincott Williams & Wilkins. Am Jrl Nur 1980;80(3):485–8. Available at: http://www.jstor.org/stable/3469921. Accessed November 11, 2011.
13. American Nurse Credentialing Center APRN Corner: Frequently asked questions. 2012. Available at: http://www.nursecredentialing.org/Certification/APRNCorner/APRN-FAQ.aspx#17. Accessed March 16, 2012.

The Future of the Population-Focused, Public Health Clinical Nurse Specialist

Dawn Doutrich, PhD, RN, CNS[a],*, Jo Ann Walsh Dotson, PhD, RN[b]

KEYWORDS

- Clinical nurse specialist • Public health • LACE population categories
- Advanced practice registered nurse • Population-focus

KEY POINTS

- Advanced practice community and public health nurse specialists possess specialized knowledge on the family and individuals across the life span.
- It is critical that we retain and promote certification examinations which allow advanced public health/community/population-focused nurses to be board certified.
- Certification of a clinical nurse specialist for the individual/family across the life span and community with a focus on public health nursing should be explored.

The purpose of this article is to address the need for continued certification of community and public health nurses at the advanced practice registered nurse (APRN) level, and to explore curricular avenues and policy recommendations with regard to certification and education of these nurses. The transformation of health care and burgeoning access to information has changed what the public expects and needs from health professionals. Nursing roles have expanded and transformed, in turn requiring that the education, licensure, certification, and accreditation of the professional likewise change. A plethora of policy documents and guiding papers relevant to graduate education in nursing and to APRN licensure and certification summarize, direct, and guide nurses and educators. Some of those documents are listed in **Table 1**.

Since this paper was submitted for publication, the Quad Council has initiated a nationwide survey of public health nurses related to certification and launched "All Out for Excellence: Certification and Degree completion for PHNs," a campaign to encourage certification. Findings of that survey and the campaign are not reflected in this article, but the authors are hopeful that certification options will be retained.

[a] College of Nursing, Washington State University, 14204 Northeast Salmon Creek Avenue, Vancouver, WA 98686, USA
[b] College of Nursing, Washington State University, PO Box 1495, Spokane, WA 99210-1495, USA
* Corresponding author.
E-mail address: Doutrich@vancouver.wsu.edu

DEFINITIONS

Advanced practice implies a higher level of expertise attributable not only to experience but also to education in a particular field. Advanced practice registered nurses (APRNs) have been defined as registered nurses who have education beyond a basic nursing education and who are certified at the national level by a recognized professional organization in a nursing specialty or at the state level, based on criteria established by a state Board of Nursing.[1] There is general agreement that recognized APRN roles are the certified nurse midwife (CNM), the certified registered nurse anesthetist (CRNA), the certified nurse practitioner (CNP), and the clinical nurse specialist (CNS).[2,3]

CNS practice is conceptualized as core competencies in 3 interacting domains called spheres of influence: those of the patient/client, nurses and nursing practices, and organizations and systems.[4] Advanced practice nursing historically has included the population-based, community, and public health clinical nurse specialist. Masters and/or doctorally prepared graduates of public health or advanced population health nursing whose programs met curricular requirements were eligible to sit for the national examination and able to be certified as CNSs. The patient/client domain for the CNS role was considered the population or community.[5]

ADVANCED COMMUNITY, POPULATION, OR PUBLIC HEALTH DESIGNATION?

There is no agreement among the community, population, or public health advanced registered practice nurses about the proper name for the role. Regardless of the title, public and community health nurses focus on population outcomes. The Association for Community Health Nurse Educators (ACHNE) state "the specialty emphasizes the title Public Health Nursing."[6(p6)] With nursing practice moving from acute care institutions to increased care practiced in the community, there needed to be a distinction made between nurses practicing in the community and nurses whose focus was the community or a population. In her classic article, Williams claimed the Public Health designation indicated a practice that was "community-based and population focused."[7(p247)] Public Health advanced practice may be considered a subset of community health nursing with advanced education in public health sciences.[6] Moreover, while there has been a push for labeling and credentialing as advanced practice public health nurses, there remain graduate programs claiming the broader population or community health classification. What is clear is that these designations do

Table 1 Policy documents and guiding papers relevant to graduate education in nursing and to ARPN licensure and certification	
Document Title	**Year Published**
American Association of Colleges of Nursing (AACN) Essentials of Masters Education in Nursing	2011
AACN Essentials of Doctoral Education for Advanced Nursing Practice (DNP)	2006
Association of Community Health Nurse Educators (ACHNE) Crossroads for Graduate Education	2007
The Consensus Model for APRN: Licensure, Accreditation, Certification & Education (LACE)	2008
Institute of Medicine's Future of Nursing: Leading Change Advancing Health	2011

not imply a specialty based on where care occurs. Instead, no matter what the label, they denote an advanced practice based on specialty sciences focused on improving populations' health, and informed by the social justice foundations of public health.

THE COMMUNITY CNS ROLE: IMPROVING POPULATION HEALTH

In the past, nurses with master's degrees in community or public health nursing have found a niche within the community/public health CNS role.[8,9] Logan[8] surveyed the 209 CNSs certified in Community Health by the American Nurses Credentialing Center (ANCC) with a response from 111 of these individuals, and found that 35% described themselves as educator; 22% defined their roles as administrator/leader; 21% were clinicians; 14% considered themselves consultants; and 8% described themselves as researchers. Logan concluded that the Community Health CNS was a viable, sought after, and satisfying professional certification. Implications were that schools of nursing should continue to offer the specialty, with more emphasis on the CNS's 3 "spheres of influence."

Most of Logan's CNS responders were not working in the public health arena; rather, 41% of these CNSs reported their primary job title to be professor, instructor, faculty, or administrator of a nursing program. Other titles included "disease intervention specialist, executive director of hospice, Community Health nurse epidemiologist, HIV clinical specialist, home health administrator, public health program manager, coordinator of cardiac education, health advocate, consultant, occupational health nurse, school nurse, and diabetes APN."[8(p46)] It is important to recall that public health workplaces rarely remunerate for certification, whereas certification may be valued in an educational or institutional role.

Acknowledging "nurses with master's degrees in community/public health nursing have advanced knowledge and skills to manage the health of populations and communities,"[(p250)] Robertson and Baldwin[9] conducted a qualitative study designed to describe the role of the advanced practice community/public health nurse specialist (C/PHNS). Their purposive sample of 10 nurses were working in a variety of community health settings, and were both interviewed and observed. Practice settings for their sample included "local and state health departments, visiting nurses associations, schools, and charitable health-related associations. Job positions included school nurse, case manager, consultant, program manager, and administrator."[9(p251)]

Robertson's and Baldwin's participants, like Logan's, described a variety of practice sites that were not easily lumped into traditional "public health" settings. Their findings included 6 advanced practice role characteristics for these participants including leadership, management, consultation, partnership building, large-scale program planning, and advocacy and policy setting. In addition, a big-picture perspective of practice was an overarching theme in all role categories. One of their participants put it this way:

...Having advanced practice nurses in the community is a role that nursing cannot value enough. I don't think that nurses appreciate how important [this role is]— after all, nursing began in the community. ...The impact that an [advanced practice] community health nurse makes in the community is not episodic. It's population based and I don't think we value enough the fact that if you stop disease transmission in 4 people you've affected 25,000 lives.[9(p254)]

The Institute of Medicine (IOM) *Future of Nursing: Leading Change, Advancing Health* (with more than 100 references to "population" in the body of the work)[10] and the American Association of Colleges of Nursing (AACN) Essentials[11,12] plainly point out the importance of understanding population health. Yet the national conversation has missed the advanced practice characteristics of "high level leadership and sophisticated advocacy and policy setting activities at the organizational, community, and state levels"[9(p254)] that these individuals embody. There seems an assumption that these characteristics, specialized knowledge, and skill sets can be inserted into non–population health APRN curricula. Certainly there must be more emphasis on prevention and maintaining population health in all APRN roles and specialties. However, without intentionality and the expertise of advanced practice in population health nursing, there is concern that the deep knowledge that results in "sophisticated advocacy" and programmatic interventions based on community assessment and big-picture upstream thinking will be lost. After the studies by Logan and Robertson and Baldwin, the ANCC's Clinical Specialist in Community/Public Health Examination was retired and replaced by the Advanced Public Health-Board Certified designation (APHN-BC).

Local public health departments have lost funding and positions over the past years. Moreover, professional nurse positions are among those that have been curtailed. While the Association of Community Health Nurse Educator's report includes discussion about the shortage of public health nurse positions and qualified faculty to teach them,[6] there is also a trend away from hiring nurses as leaders in public health. Moreover, when public health moved away from delivering primary care to the core functions model, the main work was considered to be assessment, policy development, and assurance. In this reconceptualization of public health practice and principal responsibilities, nurse clinician positions were lost. Furthermore, unlike some other APRN roles, the public health hiring market rarely remunerates advanced practice public health nurses for advanced practice certification, resulting in few public health nurses pursuing it. On the other hand, students who have graduated from community or population-focused masters, who want to work as CNSs in a specific population unit or as educators in academia or in clinical practice, want and need the certification and may be rewarded for it. Whether certification is remunerated in Public Health or not, many graduates of advanced population health programs want the added recognition that comes with the ARPN licensure, and many private institutions do value the certification and require it for certain positions.

EDUCATION AND LICENSURE FOR ALL ADVANCED PRACTICE REGISTERED NURSES

There have been numerous efforts to clarify the education, designation, and roles of APRNs. One of the most extensive and far reaching was a consensus process, which was designed initially with funding from the Division of Nursing in the Bureau of Health Professions, Health Resources and Services Administration, US Department of Health and Human Services; the consensus process is described in the final report. The process was used to assure broad and meaningful input by nursing organizations and partner organizations, and included a series of meetings beginning in 2003. The process culminated in a proposal titled "The Consensus Model for APRN: Licensure, Accreditation, Certification & Education," which was published in July 2008.[2] The model defines advanced nursing practice, describes specialty areas and titles, and proposes a regulatory model for advanced practice registered nurses, linking the efforts of state licensing boards, accrediting and certifying bodies, and educational organizations.[2] The Licensure, Accreditation, Certification and Education (LACE) model requires that in addition to receiving education for a particular role (CNM, CRNA, CNS, and CNP), APRN students must also receive education focusing on at least 1 of 6 populations: family/individual across the life span, adult-gerontology, pediatrics, neonatal, women's health/gender-related, or psychiatric/mental health. Course work must also include 3 "separate graduate-level courses in advanced physiology/pathophysiology, health assessment and pharmacology"[2(p5)] along with a minimum of 500 hours of related clinical experiences. Educational programs offering advanced nursing education study are to be accredited, meaning their graduates are eligible for national specialty certification, and included within graduate programs that are also accredited.

The Quad Council of Public Health Nursing Organizations is comprised of the Association of State and Territorial Directors of Nursing (ASTDN), the American Nurses Association Council on Nursing Practice and Economics (ANA), the ACHNE, and the Section of Public Health Nursing of the American Public Health Association (APHA). Eleven individuals from these 4 organizations provide leadership and are charged with promoting public health/community health nursing. Levin and colleagues[6] describe the Quad Council representatives' participation (2 years after the process began) in the development of the Consensus document. The major proposal the Quad Council offered, an alternative definition of advanced practice that would not limit it to "the direct care of individuals or to the use of pharmacologic interventions,"[6(p10)] was rejected by the APRN workgroup.

Essentials of Master's Education and the LACE Document

Despite the efforts of the APRN workgroup to clarify and standardize advanced practice nursing education, nurses, partner health professionals, and the public continue to be confused about the definition of, practice settings for, and education of APRNs. The questions surrounding the role and functions of APRNs are perhaps most perplexing in the advanced population and public health arena. Many of the documents outlining educational and practice expectations of APRNs appear to recognize incongruities between public health and other advanced practice roles, often "exempting" public health in some fashion. For example, the LACE document describes the CNS as responsible for diagnosis and treatment of "health/illness states, disease management, health promotion, and prevention of illness and risk behaviors among individuals, families, groups, and communities."[2(p9)] Health promotion and disease prevention in families, groups, and communities is the role of public health nursing, therefore the role of the CNS with focus on the family/individual across the life-span population group seems a precise definition of the ARPN practicing in many population and public health settings. Ervin[5] notes that "to maintain or enhance the health of a community, often interventions are performed at the individual level, such as immunizations. Care at the individual level is not a negation of the community focus but part of the total scope of practice needed to achieve healthy communities."[5(p218)]

The LACE document states that nurses practicing in roles and specialties that do not provide "direct care to individuals" do NOT require "regulatory recognition beyond the Registered Nurse license."[2(p9)] Public health and advanced practice population health nurses may function as leaders in local and state public health settings, directing and implementing policy decisions affecting the health of communities; or they may be in leadership positions in health care systems with responsibilities for many hundreds of patients. Unfortunately, the LACE document indicates that nurses providing "indirect" or population-based care may not use the designation of ARPN, or other role titles that may "confuse the public." Nevertheless, these certifications may be sought by the individual nurse graduate or be required by the employer for the population health CNS, especially outside of traditional public health settings.

If public health or other population-focused nurses participate in a course of study that includes advanced pathophysiology, advanced physical assessment, and advanced pharmacology (the 3 Ps), specialized content regarding public health theory and practice and the required clinical experience hours, and are accredited by national organizations, it is appropriate that the designation of CNS be accorded them, as it is to other ARPNs. Confusion arose with the recent publication (March 2011) of the *Essentials of Master's Education in Nursing*. This document, developed and published by the American Association of College of Nurses, "delineates the graduate nursing core competencies for all master's graduates."[12(p7)] Despite the inclusive intent, two sets of competencies are described; one for master's graduates with "indirect care practice roles" and a second for those assuming "direct care roles."[12(p8)] The definitions of direct and indirect included in the glossary are imprecise and open to interpretation, but the implication, that master's programs preparing students for "direct care" must assure that students complete "three separate comprehensive, graduate courses," has far-reaching implications on advanced nursing education. Schools of nursing across the United States are trying to interpret this requirement so that they can modify or create courses, change curricular guidelines, and seek university approvals to assure that they will be ready for the 2015 implementation date.

Implications for Advanced Practice Population and Public Health Nursing

A challenge identified in part in the LACE model is the requirement that APRNs be vetted in the form of an Accredited Certification Program offering a certification process or examination. At present, the American Board of Nursing Specialties (ABNS) and the National Commission for Certifying Agencies (NCAA) recognize the ANCC which certifies Advanced Public Health Nurses.[13] Currently, nurses who have completed graduate education in public or community health nursing at a graduate program with a clinical nurse specialist program that includes three separate advanced courses in pathophysiology, pharmacology, and health assessment as well as a minimum of 500 clinical hours may request that the PHCNS-BC, a clinical nurse specialist credential, be awarded, instead of the APHN-BC.[14] In part because of the limited number of registrants sitting for the advanced public health examination, there have been rumors that the examination may be canceled. The LACE model incorporates certification as evidence of mastery; if the certification examination is discontinued, advanced community and public health nurse specialists will not have a certification process as required in the LACE model.

The definitions of direct and indirect care are indistinct at best, and may be disregarded by some, but the fact that advanced practice public health nurses are not required to take coursework required by all other advanced practice roles seems to be, at best, shortsighted. Rather than excuse public or population health nurses from taking the 3 Ps, this is a time to incorporate population content into all courses and increase the rigor and status of the specialty. Understanding that the request for excusing advanced public health or community specialists from the 3 Ps came in part from the public health community, and that the AACN Essentials and the Consensus (LACE) document were crafted in part in response to the outcry from public health practitioners, does not mean that the outcome serves the nation well. In fact there is a rethink taking place among some public health leaders. Sarah Abrams, editor of *Public Health Nursing*, states that she

> *...cannot get hot and bothered about whether the so called 3 Ps are required. Nurses are nurses, even if they practice at the population level. The public expects us to know anatomy and physiology; they have every right to expect us to*

understand pharmacology and how to conduct a physical examination. It only enhances credibility when we talk about health promotion and disease prevention to be able to discuss the physiologic impact of disease or the inappropriate use of certain pharmaceuticals.[15(p314)]

This statement comes at a time when the IOM Future of Nursing is emphasizing the importance of population-based health promotion and disease prevention, and when the United States is struggling to reform the health care system and emphasize prevention. The ACHNE Crossroads report identified critical content areas for advanced practice nurses including, but not limited to, those in the public health arena.[6] The IOM report and the AACN's Essentials for Master's and Doctoral Education also state that advanced practice nursing education includes the same critical content areas identified in the Crossroads report, including population-centered nursing theory, interdisciplinary practice, leadership and systems thinking, biostatistics, epidemiology, and health policy for all advanced practice nurses, not just public health.[11] Acknowledging those specialized role characteristics, knowledge, and skill sets identified by Robertson and Baldwin, public and community health nurses need to be able to continue to pursue advanced practice degrees to develop a wide-ranging and thorough depth of knowledge regarding systems theory, epidemiology, biostatistics, and health policy development aimed at reinventing the health care system.[9]

The Essentials of Doctoral Education for Advanced Nursing Practice

The Doctor of Nursing Practice (DNP) is the preferred degree for specialized advanced practice nursing. As more and more schools of nursing transition to these advanced practice degree requirements and more certifying and credentialing bodies make this change, population and public health advanced practice programs will need to ensure inclusion. The ANCC Master's Essentials make clear that graduate public health nurses can be prepared at the master's level, yet there is a need for the kind of leadership and expertise the DNP promises in the area of population health. The ACHNE Crossroads document includes curricular guidance for doctoral advanced population and public health programs, and supports the "national movement toward the DNP as a terminal degree for advanced nursing practice."[6(p17)]

RECOMMENDATIONS RELATED TO CURRICULA AND POLICY

Nursing and nurse leaders must assume responsibility to implement the LACE model while also assuring that graduate nurses enter the workforce able to address the health care needs of the population. The LACE document allows that "new specialties emerge based on health needs of the population."[2(p11)] Although the advanced population and public health specialist is not a new role, it is one geared to well address the needs of the population.[2]

The Future of Nursing report emphasizes the importance of using nurses to the full extent of their education and the importance of integrating population-based information in all curricula. The complex and sophisticated specialist knowledge and experience held by advanced practice population-focused, community, and public health nurses must be honored.

The distinction between direct and indirect nursing does not serve the profession or the nation's health needs well. The Master's Essentials document distinguishes between the provision of direct and indirect care by nurses, defining direct care as "… nursing care provided to individuals or families that is intended to achieve specific health goals"[12(p33)] or outcomes that can be delivered in a variety of settings. Indirect care is defined as "...nursing decisions, actions, or interventions that are provided through or on behalf of individuals, families, or groups."[12(p33)] The distinction between these types of care is imprecise and creates artificial distinctions that are not useful, and in fact create factions within the profession that should not exist.

Given the current context of public health whereby nurses are becoming scarcer and there is little support for certification, the advanced practice population health CNS may be located outside the typical public health setting, at least until more dollars and status move to public health. Therefore, it is useful to continue to label the advanced practice role broadly, to include population health, public health, and community health, while understanding that community is a conceptual designation rather than where practice takes place. This broad labeling is in response to the need for population-focused nurses in multiple sites and the current, unfortunate lack of remuneration for advanced certification in public health nursing. Having the option of being certified as a CNS in this important specialty is crucial. The certification opportunity helps to keep the graduate programs viable, and ensures the advanced population practice based on public health sciences.

In addition, most advanced practice community and public health nurse specialists possess specialized knowledge on the family/individual across the life span. This population focus is one of the 6 LACE population categories. At present, there exists no CNS certifying examination that would capture the advanced population health graduate with this population focus. Exploring the need for and marketability of this certification is urged. The institution of a CNS certification for the individual/family across the life-span population focus, inclusive of the advanced population health understanding of the community and public health nurse, could answer the need for a clinical nurse specialist without the direct/indirect schism. Finally, it is critical for nurse educators and certifying bodies to assure that all APRNs receive graduate-level education in physical assessment, physiology, pharmacology, epidemiology, biostatistics, and population-based intervention approaches. Through understanding these core areas, APRNs can better serve the nation's complex and increasing health needs.

REFERENCES

1. Mosby. Mosby's medical dictionary. 8th edition. Mosby; 2009.
2. National Council of State Boards of Nursing. Consensus model on APRN regulation: licensure, accreditation, certification, and education. APRN consensus work group & NCSBN APRN advisory committee. National Council of State Boards of Nursing; 2008. Available at: http://www.aacn.nche.edu/education-resources/APRNReport.pdf. Accessed October 27, 2011.
3. O'Grady E. Advanced practice registered nurses: the impact on patient safety and quality. In: Hughes RG, editor. Patient safety and quality: an evidence-based handbook for nurses. Rockville (MD): Agency for Healthcare Research and Quality; 2008. p. 1126–45.
4. Fulton B. Evolution of clinical nurse specialist role and practice in the United States. In: Fulton B, Lyon B, Goudreau K, editors. Foundations of clinical nurse specialist practice. New York: Springer Publishing Company; 2010. p. 3–13.
5. Ervin N. Community as client: clinical nurse specialist role. In: Fulton B, Lyon B, Goudreau K, editors. Foundations of clinical nurse specialist practice. New York: Springer Publishing Company; 2010. p. 213–21.
6. Levin P, Cary A, Kulbok P, et al. Association of Community Health Nurse Educators Task Force on Graduate Education for Advanced Practice. Graduate education for

advanced practice public health nursing: at the crossroads. Public Health Nurs 2008;25(2):176–93.

7. Williams CA. Community-based population-focused practice: the foundation of specialization in public health practice. In: Stanhope M, Lancaster J, editors. Community health nursing: process and practice of promoting health. St Louis (MO): Mosby; 1992.

8. Logan L. The practice of certified community health CNSs. Clin Nurse Spec 2005; 19(1):43–8.

9. Robertson JF, Baldwin KB. Advanced practice role characteristics of the community/public health nurse specialist. Clin Nurse Spec 2007;21(5):250–4.

10. IOM, the future of nursing: leading change, advancing health. Washington, DC: National Academies Press; 2011.

11. AACN, The essentials of doctoral education for advanced nursing practice. 2006. Available at: http://www.aacn.nche.edu/publications/position/dnpessentials.pdf. Accessed October 26, 2011.

12. The essentials of master's education in nursing. AACN; 2011. Available at: http://www.aacn.nche.edu/education-resources/MastersEssentials11.pdf. Accessed October 26, 2011.

13. ANCC. Public health nurse, advanced. 2011 [cited; credentialing process, and criteria]. Available at: http://www.nursecredentialing.org/Certification/NurseSpecialties/AdvPublicHealth.aspx. Accessed October 26, 2011.

14. ANCC. Advanced public health nursing 2011 testing information/certification application form. Available at: http://www.nursecredentialing.org/Documents/Certification/Application/NursingSpecialty/PublicHealthNursingAdvancedApplication.aspx. Accessed October 26, 2011.

15. Abrams SA. Credentials, skills, and recognition. Public Health Nurs 2010;27(5): 383–4.

Erratum

In the March 2012 issue of Nursing Clinics of North America, an error was made in the article, "E-cigarettes: Promise or Peril." Reference number 37 contained a misspelling of the author's name. The correct spelling of the author's name in reference 37 is "Caponnetto."

We apologize for this oversight.

Nurs Clin N Am 47 (2012) 315
doi:10.1016/j.cnur.2012.04.003
0029-6465/12/$ – see front matter © 2012 Elsevier Inc. All rights reserved.

Index

Note: Page numbers of article titles are in **boldface** type.

A

Academic Center for Evidence-Based Practice (ACE), ACE Star Model for advanced-practice registered nursing, 269–270
Accreditation, in Consensus Model for APRN Regulation, 247
Accreditation Commission for Midwifery Education, 210–211
Acute care, future practice of nurse practitioners in, 185–186
Advanced practice registered nurses (APRNs), future of, 181–313
    certified nurse midwives, **205–213**
    certified registered nurse anesthetists, **215–223**
    clinical nurse specialists, **193–203**
    doctorate in nursing practice, **225–240**
    impact of interprofessional collaboration, **283–294**
    impact of new regulatory standards on practice of, **241–250**
    IOM quality reports and implications for, **251–260**
    nurse practitioners, **181–191**
    population-focused public health clinical nurse specialists, **305–313**
    psychiatric mental health clinical nurse specialists, **295–304**
    role in ensuring evidence-based practice, **269–281**
    role of nurse executive in fostering and empowering, **261–267**
Affordable Care Act. *See* Patient Protection and Affordable Care Act
American Association of Nurse Anesthetists, view on doctor of nursing practice (DNP) degree, 237
American College of Nurse-Midwives, view on doctor of nursing practice (DNP) degree, 237–238
American Midwifery Certification Board, 210–211
Anesthesia, certified registered nurse anesthetist practice, **215–223**
    educational requirements for, 219–220
    future of, 221–223
    history of, 216–217
    safe, cost-effective anesthesia care by, 218–219

C

Certification, for population-focused public health clinical nurse specialists, 308–311
    in Consensus Model for APRN Regulation, 247–248
    of psychiatric mental health clinical nurse specialists (PMHCNS), 299
Certified nurse practitioners (CNP), future of practice, **181–191**
    in acute care, 185–186
    in primary care, 184–185
    international, global, and cultural issues, 186–187
    public image, 187–188
    regulation and policy, 182–184
    world of opportunity for, 188–189

Nurs Clin N Am 47 (2012) 317–322
doi:10.1016/S0029-6465(12)00046-1
0029-6465/12/$ – see front matter © 2012 Elsevier Inc. All rights reserved.

nursing.theclinics.com

Quality (*continued*)
    Health Professions Education, 256–258
    Keeping Patients Safe, 256
    To Err is Human, 253

R

Regulations, for nurse practitioner practice, 182–184
    impact of new standards on advanced practice registered nursing, **241–250**
        Consensus Model for APRN Regulation, 242–243
            implications for all APRNs, 244–249
            Licensure, Accreditation, Certification and Education (LACE), 243–244
Reimbursement, for APRN services, impact of interprofessional collaboration on, 288–289

S

Safety, of certified registered nurse anesthetist practice, 218–219
Safety, patient, IOM report on, 256
Standards. *See* Regulations.

W

Women's health, nurse-midwifery, **205–213**

Moving?

Make sure your subscription moves with you!

To notify us of your new address, find your **Clinics Account Number** (located on your mailing label above your name), and contact customer service at:

Email: journalscustomerservice-usa@elsevier.com

800-654-2452 (subscribers in the U.S. & Canada)
314-447-8871 (subscribers outside of the U.S. & Canada)

Fax number: 314-447-8029

Elsevier Health Sciences Division
Subscription Customer Service
3251 Riverport Lane
Maryland Heights, MO 63043